Caring for Someone in Your Home

K.N. Tigges

W.M. Marcil

C.J. Alterio

Additional copies of this book may be ordered through bookstores or by
sending $11.95 plus $2.75 for postage and handling to:
Publishers Distribution Service
121 East Front Street, Suite 203
Traverse City, MI 49684

Copyright © 1992 by MAST Health Group
Published by: MAST Health Group: 93 Highgate Avenue, Buffalo, NY 14214

To the best of our knowledge, the procedures described in this
publication reflect currently accepted practice; nevertheless, they
cannot be considered absolute and universal recommendations.
All recommendations must be considered in light of the individual's
condition and care and in light of any new information that has
become available since the publishing of this text. The authors and
the publisher disclaim responsibility and assume no liability for
any adverse effects resulting directly or indirectly from the suggested procedures, from any undetected errors, or from the
reader's misunderstanding of the text.

The authors and publisher suggest that each individual check
with their physician for specific application of these techniques to
their individual situation before using them.

Publisher's Cataloging-in-Publication Data
Tigges, K.N.,
        Caring for someone in your home / K.N. Tigges, W.M. Marcil, C.J.
    Alterio. – [S.1.] : MAST Health Group, 1992.
        p. : ill. ; cm.
        Spine title: Caring. Includes index.
        ISBN 0-9633017-0-5
        1. Physically handicapped – Home care – Handbooks, manuals, etc.
        2. Aged – Home care – Handbooks, manuals, etc. 3. Home nursing.
        4. Home care services – United States. I. Marcil, W.M.
        II. Alterio, C.J. III. Title. IV. Title: Caring.
        RT61.T54   1992

        649.8-dc20   92-81466
                        SLS92-96

Manufactured in the United States of America.

About This Book

Home health care in America is rapidly growing. More and more patients, families, and significant others, have to learn how to manage medical problems, how to provide physical and personal care, and how to go on living day-to-day.

For many, being at home, or caring for someone in your home is most desirable. However, it requires learning many new skills and making major adjustments in lifestyle. The authors and contributors of this book have, collectively, over 130 years of experience in working with the physically ill, disabled, and their family members in hospitals, rehabilitation centers, and homes, both rural and urban. They appreciate as much as you do the concerns, worries, and frustrations of having to learn so many new skills.

This book is intended to help ease some of the frustrations that may be encountered. It does not intend to be complete, or to address all problems, concerns, or situations that may arise. We do hope that what we present will provide you with some help — some direction — some support — some guidance — some encouragement.

Authors

Kent Nelson Tigges, MS, OTR, FAOTA, FHIH, is Associate Professor of Occupational Therapy at the University at Buffalo, State University of New York, and is involved in private practice in home health care, including hospice care.

William Matthew Marcil, MS, OTR, is a consulting occupational therapist in private practice in Virginia Beach, Virginia. He has extensive experience in acute care, long-term care, rehabilitation and hospice care programs. He currently specializes in home health care in Tidewater, Virginia.

Christopher John Alterio, OTR, was formerly in private practice in rural New York. Presently he is the Director of Occupational Therapy at the Rehabilitation Center in Allegany, New York. He is experienced in post-acute, long-term, and hospice home care for children and adults with physical, psychiatric, and developmental disabilities.

Contributing Authors

Rose Causley, Chapter 2.

J. Robert Davis, Sr., BS (Pharm), Chapter 5.

Leah Hoover, MS, RN, Chapter 8.

Kathleen Hutton, LPN, COTA, Chapter 6.

Mary Langstaff, MN, RN, Chapter 3.

Acknowledgments

Word processing of this manuscript by Jacquelyn Rankin, Department of Occupational Therapy, University at Buffalo, State University of New York.

Illustrations by David Maas, MA, and John Joseph Mullins.

Design, production, and proofreading by Michael Alterio.

Cover streetscape taken from "Five Houses in Buffalo" by Ray Hassard. Photograph courtesy of Ray Hassard. Cover artwork by Educational Technology Services, SUNY Buffalo and Donald Watkins and Catherine Ohki.

Contents

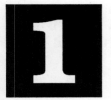

A Disabled Person's Message to Others

When the authors of this text first asked me to write a section for their book I was very flattered. Then I thought about it and decided that "my story" about my illness and resulting disability would not be of much or any interest or value to anyone else. The more I thought about it, the more I began to think about my life, my relationship with my family, friends, and co-workers, and perhaps more importantly, about their relationships with me since I have become disabled. Although my illness and disability, and its implications, are very specifically personal to me, I began to think that there are perhaps many common threads of feelings and concerns that we all share, so I decided what I have experienced may be of some value or interest to others. Perhaps, if we talk about it together, we can learn together and find some comfort and strength from our experiences — and hopefully some courage to better face ourselves and those we love and care about tomorrow, and for the weeks and months to come.

I have always thought of myself as a reasonably responsible, hard-working person. I worked hard, cared for, and looked after my family — I know you did also. My work brought me into contact daily with sick, ill, and disabled people. In the past 40 years, I have treated many people and their families. I have seen much heartache, pain, anguish, disappointment, anger, resentment, and frustration. I have seen some people and their family members crumble and be destroyed. I have also seen people, despite great adversities, rise up from their adversity and build new and productive lives.

Many times I thought that my experiences would be of great help should something serious happen in my life. Somehow I thought that I would be better prepared to cope. Believe me, none of my experiences helped at all. It is all very different when one is on the other side of the fence. No matter what some people may say, it is impossible to prepare, no matter how much or little experience or education you have had. So you must not feel guilty or inadequate or irresponsible when you experience a life crisis. It's okay to not be brave, or to not know or do or say, all the right things.

I know that most of us didn't think very much about being seriously ill or disabled, although we know others that it has happened to. We hoped and prayed that it wouldn't ever happen to us, or anyone else we loved or cared about. When I was rushed to the hospital in an ambulance, although I was scared to death, it never crossed my mind that whatever it was that was happening to me would be permanent and would change my life substantially.

When I was in the hospital, good and caring people took care of me. They took over, as they must do. As a result, I lost all measures of control. They told me what I had to do — what I could not do, what I could do. I know they were right and that they meant well, but somewhere in this process I was lost. I became the stroke in Room 44, Bed 2. They didn't know who I was and that I was frightened about all that was happening to me.

A good friend of mine once said to me when her daughter was critically ill in the hospital that "somehow you feel that you must be good and totally cooperative. That you mustn't ask too many questions, or disagree with all those clever professionals, for if you do, they might think you to be a troublemaker, and hold you to blame if things didn't work out as they had scheduled." At the time I thought she was overreacting, but now

I know exactly how she felt. All these "clever" people take over. "Do this, don't do this." "You are only making things worse for yourself." "You could be worse, you could be like the patient in the next bed." "I know just how you are feeling." And those therapists! I wonder how many of them have ever tried to imagine what it would be like to be in my place. They set goals without even asking me what it is that I need to do to survive today, tomorrow, and for the years to come. There was only one occupational therapist that even ventured to ask me who I was, what I did in life, and what I wanted to get out of this disastrous situation. To this day I treasure his honesty and straightforwardness. Please don't get me wrong. They were all very nice people, they were friendly, and I know that they were truly concerned with my health. But let's be honest and realistic with each other. Perhaps they do know some things that should or should not be done — let's give them some credit — but they should take some lessons from us, or at least try to empathize with us before they present their categorical "do's" and "don't's". God, how tired and frustrated I got from being given advice, being scolded. I do know that they all meant well, but please give me some credit — I'm not completely stupid. Just because I don't show you my feelings and concerns doesn't mean that I don't have them.

This brings me to the issue of isolation. How well I remember all those staff conversations with, and without, my family members present. I wonder if hospital personnel stop to think that patients have nothing to do, the majority of the time they spend in the hospital, except to watch and listen. As most of us are not completely deaf, we listen with careful attention to what is being said. Hushed voices in corridors carry well. If you have something to say about me, my care, my future, or what is going to happen to or be done to me, please say it openly and honestly to me. You do me no favors by pretending that I do not know or need to know how sick or disabled I am. This goes also for my family members. Please do not suggest to, or threaten, the hospital staff to not tell me what is going on. Your well-intentioned thoughts become lies and will only strain our relationship. More than ever, now is the time when we must be honest and realistic with each other so that we can set realistic and appropriate plans and goals for tomorrow and the future.

When I was being discharged, the nurse brought all my medicine in to me in a white paper bag. She went over each one with me and then put them into my suitcase. When she walked out of the room, I couldn't remember a thing she had said, my mind was a total blur. At the time I didn't worry about it, as I knew all I needed to do was to read the labels on the pill bottles. Then the hospital discharge planner came in and said everything was set for me to go home. She said that a wheelchair, walker, commode and hospital bed would be delivered to my home before the end of the day. She reminded me that the occupational therapist had taught me how to use the equipment and that the transition from the hospital to home would go smoothly.

The thought of going home brought mixed feelings. On one hand I wanted to go home in the worst way, as at long last I could sleep in my own bed, be with my family, and that I would be safe and secure, and that, at long last, life would be normal again! On the other hand, the thought of leaving the hospital brought me some anxiety. For so long these doctors, nurses, and therapists were watching over and taking care of me. Looking back I hadn't realized how safe and secure their care and attention had made me feel. I really had felt safe. It was so reassuring to me that as long as I was in the hospital nothing would happen to me, and if it did, they would be right there to take care of whatever happened. Now I wish that I had not been so grumpy and difficult at times. You know sometimes we don't see things clearly or realistically when we are scared, hurt, or under great stress.

When the ambulance drove into my driveway, I couldn't believe I was really home at last. How good it was going to be to crawl into my own bed. The ambulance drivers carried me upstairs on a stretcher and into my room. The first thing that caught my eye was a shiny hospital bed where my familiar old bed used to be. It was at that moment that I knew somehow that everything was not going to be the same. Starting life at home again was no easy task. Trying to establish a new routine was a nightmare filled with frustration. The thrill of being home quickly became a mixed blessing. I couldn't get out of bed without help. The wheelchair would not go through the bathroom door. Having to sit on a commode with someone watching me was humiliating, to say the least. The days became very long as I was confined to the upstairs. My world shrunk to the walls of my bedroom. One day I decided to become adventuresome. I wheeled my wheelchair to the bathroom door and carefully stood up and made my way to the toilet. As I sat there the sense of accomplishment was great. I thought to myself, "I can do something after all. I'm not completely helpless." I then heard someone coming up the steps. When they saw me all hell broke loose. A tirade of, "What are you doing, why didn't you call me, you could have fallen and hit your head, broken your hip, don't ever do this again, I'd never forgive myself if something happened to you!" When one is attacked, it is normal to defend, so I let loose. I said some terrible things like, "If I have to live my life like this, I'd rather be dead." Of course I didn't really mean it, but the frustration of not being able or permitted to do even the most basic things panicked me. Then there were tears, requests for forgiveness, and promises to be good.

The next day, one of those Fisher Price baby monitors was put on my bedside table. You know what these things are, don't you? They are "bugs" — listening devices. They use them in the spy movies to listen to what people are saying and doing. The irony of this situation was that, when I was practicing my profession, I frequently recommended these monitors to family members because I knew how they would worry for fear their loved one would fall out of bed, or need something and they wouldn't know it unless they were close by. Family members have to go on living their lives also, and they can't be expected to be within ear reach twenty-four hours a day. Funny enough it had never crossed my mind, until now, how the patient might have felt to lose all privacy. In order to retrieve some privacy, I quickly discovered that by putting the corner of the bedspread over the "bug" I could move around the room without someone running up the stairs and checking on me. The sixth and seventh steps from the top of the stairway squeak, so I always had plenty of time to remove the bedspread before someone arrived in the doorway. I would pretend to be surprised to see them, and say, "Is there something you wanted?" This little charade brought me not only some amusement, but also something to do besides stare at the walls all day.

Much of the time in the weeks that followed I spent a lot of time day-dreaming, reminiscing about the past. It helped a great deal in ultimately letting go of the person I once was. One is what one has done in life. Each of us is made up of our past life experiences, and to do differently now than in the past is to become a different person, and that is a very difficult thing to do. Age and life experiences have little to do with it. It purely depends on the way in which you viewed and valued your life and what you did with it before the disability reared its ugly head and destroyed all your plans for the future.

Someone once wrote that one's work is the single greatest index of a person's worth and value to society, and that by making a contribution to life, one gains respect for oneself and the admiration of others. Whoever said this was absolutely correct. By our very nature, we are active and productive people, and no matter how small or great our contributions may have been, we made them, and a personal sense of pride and accomplishment was what made us get up in the morning and face our responsibilities. To wake up in the morning knowing that there are no productive plans, no goals to work on, and no contribution to make, is perhaps the worst death sentence one can receive in life.

In the next couple pages I would like to share with you some of my thoughts on how to work through some of these concerns, dilemmas, and frustrations.

To the person with a disability:

It is absolutely normal to want to hold on to your past — to close your eyes and hope the nightmare will go away. It is perfectly normal to believe that you are still the person that you once were, even though your body doesn't do what you want it to do. It is perfectly normal to resent your family, friends, and co-workers telling you "not to worry, everything is going to work out okay —that you have worked hard all your life, take life easy now — let someone else now do the work." They mean well, and say these things out of love and concern for you. They are trying their best to ease your pain. As hard on you as it is to do, say thank you and that you appreciate their help and concern.

Above and beyond all, keep their friendship. In your relationship with your family, be patient, understanding, and appreciative of the stresses, worries, and concerns they are having. After all, you are not the only one that is struggling — so are they. Their lives have also been turned upside-down. They have no more idea than you do what they are supposed to do, or how to do it. They worry for fear that they won't remember all the right ways to take care of you — they worry themselves sick for fear that something will happen to you that they could have prevented. Even more painfully, many family members hold themselves personally responsible for what happened to you. "If I had only noticed this or that, all of this wouldn't have happened." What a ghastly sense of guilt they unnecessarily carry on their shoulders. Help them, somehow, to not feel guilty or responsible for what has happened. This is so important for all of you. As strange as it may seem, under the circumstances, it is up to you to ease their pain. As much as you are suffering, you do have a responsibility to those that love and care about you — please do not forget this, for everyone's future depends on a mutual understanding and respect for and with each other.

Slowly and gracefully let go of your past. It is not a sign of defeat to give up those things that will no longer be possible. Doing this is not an act of weakness, as you may think or feel, but rather strength. You may never have thought that you could muster up the strength to make something positive out of all of this. But believe me, you can, and you must. Redirect your anger and resentment into positive thoughts, ideas, and goals. A life of anger, bitterness, and/or disappointment is no way for any human being to live out their life no matter how long or short it may be. Start to make a list, no matter how unrealistic or impractical it may be, about what you would like to do and accomplish with your life. You know there are many options, many opportunities out there. As you know, I was initially confined to my bedroom upstairs. The home care occupational therapist suggested that we put the hospital bed in the living room on the first floor of the house. He explained that I could then be more involved in what was going on and that it would save my family members much running up and down the stairs literally hundreds of times a day. The nicest thing he did was to say that this was an option, but we as a family must decide if it would work for us. After much thought, we, together, decided that I would stay upstairs. I do know that there are many families that have decided to put the bed and necessary equipment in either the living room or dining room and that it has proved to work out very satisfactorily.

I remembered that the occupational therapist had said there were options, so I began to think. It was then that I called my son-in-law, John. I reminded him that he had said he would do anything for me, so I called him on it! We made a plan for him to come over one evening a week, or on the weekend and carry me down the stairs. You know, it didn't bother me being thrown over his shoulder like a bag of potatoes and carried down the stairs, because I had decided it was important for me to get out of my room, and the goal of being with my family, downstairs, was much more important than the means by which I got there. Perhaps, more importantly, was the fact that my son-in-law and I developed a new kind of relationship — a partnership that perhaps would never have developed otherwise. To this day, I treasure that relationship very much. I am so glad that I finally looked out of my misery and initiated a plan to do something positive.

When my family saw me smiling and laughing they began to do so also. It was at that point that we started to talk openly and honestly with each other. What a relief it was for each and every one of us. At last we were talking together as a family.

To family members:

From the first day of hospitalization through your family member's return to home, and thereafter, keep your relationships open and honest. Please don't get caught up in some sense of duty, that by protecting them from the truth of what is really happening, it will in some way make things easier for either you or them. I am well aware that good and well-meaning family members, by instinct and good intentions, will sometimes do anything to spare a family member from bad or devastating news. We have all done this at one time or another, simply because we love and care about them so very much. In the long run many of these good intentions all too frequently strain relationships beyond repair. When trust and respect are broken it is very difficult to restore them. Don't let anyone, particularly hospital professionals, influence you one way or another as to what would be best to tell your family member. The important thing to remember here is, to decide what is best for you and your family. What might be the right thing for one family may be the wrong thing for yours. Think everything through very clearly before you decide. I know that in a time of crisis it is not the best time to think clearly, so please sit down together and make a plan that you think will be the best one. If it doesn't work out as you had planned, at least you know you did the very best you could have done at the time. If you start out this way there is a greater opportunity to adjust your plans than if you start out with deception.

One of the first things that I recommend to you and your family is to realize that you can't do everything that needs to be done by yourselves. Please do not feel that you have to prove to yourself, family members, or your neighbors that you will manage no matter what. I know that you feel and believe that you must do this because of honor and responsibility to your family members. To be sure, this is one of the most honorable commitments you can make to the one you love.

One of the first things that my family and I decided was that we couldn't continue to do everything that needed to be done by ourselves. We agreed that we could all benefit from some outside help. My family and I are a middle income family, and for sure we didn't have any extra money to throw away. We started by calling local hospitals and inquiring how to obtain home health services. They were very helpful in directing us to available services. Some of the first questions they asked were what services we needed, how much our income was, and where we lived. This was all very helpful. Even though we were not certain what services we needed, we sat down and made a tentative list. For our family, it was my personal care — the bathing, dressing in the morning, getting me back to bed in the evening, and someone to stay with me a couple afternoons a week so my family could get out of the house and not worry about me being left home alone. We finally decided on a home health care agency that could provide a nurse to monitor, on a weekly basis, my physical status and medications; an occupational therapist who would teach us safe transfers in and out of bed and into my wheelchair; how to use, and what affordable equipment would make using the toilet and bathtub easy and safe; ways to get down stairs, get out doors, and to go places.

When you start looking around for a home health care program, be very particular and cautious before you make a final decision. A few questions to be sure to ask: 1) Is the agency certified? 2) Are their staff properly trained in home care services? 3) What professional services do they offer, what training have they had, and how many patients have they taken care of? Ask to see personnel references from families that their staff have cared for. No matter how impressive the agency may sound on the telephone, in person, or in your home, the proof of "advertised quality care" can only be adequately verified by their customer's evaluations. 4) When you decide on a given agency, be sure, before you sign an agreement, who is going to pay for the services. Be certain to have it in writing. Remember no matter how dependent you may become on the agency that you select, you, your health insurance, medicare, or medicaid are paying good hard-earned money for these services. If you are not satisfied with their services or the services are not meeting your particular needs, do not hesitate to call the agency and let them know your concerns. Never feel trapped into keeping a particular agency for fear that you will be left high and dry without any help. In this day and age there are many health care agencies and community services competing with each other to provide good and comprehensive care.

Now, if I may, a word to my family, and perhaps to yours. As painful as it is for me to even think about it, I know that there is a real possibility, down the road, that I may become too ill and/or disabled for you to continue to take care of me at home, or your health or ability may fail and you just can no longer provide for my needs, let alone yours. Let's face it, it is a possibility, as you and I have both seen it happen to others. If you can keep me at home, that would be wonderful, but if you can't, please do not hesitate, feel guilty, or feel that somehow you have failed. You are only capable of doing so much and for so long. The last thing in the world that I would want to happen is that something would happen to your health or happiness, even though I might forget to remind you. When the time comes that you have to make the decision to put me in a nursing home, a skilled nursing facility, or the like, please consider the following: 1) get some outside help in looking at the most appropriate and affordable placement for me. 2) If I am still lucid, have my wits about me, am reasonable and rational, please include me in the planning of this placement. I can't promise you that I will be agreeable, but in the long run I think that I would, perhaps retrospectively, appreciate the courtesy of being included. If I am particularly fond of a grandson, grand-daughter, brother/sister-in-law, life-long friend, priest, minister, rabbi, or therapist, you may consider asking them to join you when you first approach me with the idea. You know many of us often respond more rationally when bad news or a major change in life is presented either by, or in the company of, someone other than our spouse or immediate family. If I am unwilling to accept the decision, simply tell me this is the way it must be for everyone's peace of mind. Be kind but firm. 3) If I am not lucid, am unreasonable, irrational, make the decision without including me. When all the plans are put into place, simply, but with love and understanding, tell me.

All of this sounds very well and good, logical and straight-forward. What it does not say are the feelings, emotions, and conflicts that are involved for family members who have to make these decisions. I would be foolish to tell you that it is easy or straightforward. For certain it is not. But in the final analysis, you must sincerely think of your lives — your health — your happiness — your future. Yes, you will perhaps feel guilty, and that is allowed for a while. Guilt is a very real feeling when one has to make a decision to make a major separation with one that one cares about.

The dilemma of not knowing what is the right thing to do can be extremely emotionally and physically draining. When you are torn — uncertain about the future — decisions and goals cannot be formulated or plans put into place. Such uncertainty can lead to strained interpersonal relationships between family members, and this is certainly no time for that to happen. Should this situation occur for you, you may want to consider the following. Take a piece of paper and a pen, and at the top of the paper write: Decision: place mom/dad in a nursing home. Then make a list of the concrete/realistic reasons why this decision should be made. List the advantages and disadvantages of your decision. Then list those family members that will support/not support your decision. When you have finished your list, fold it up, put it in an envelope, and put it in a safe place. Go on about your usual routine, and in about a week, get it out and look it over. Make any changes — add/delete, then put it away again. Then take out a second piece of paper and write: Decision: keep mom/dad at home. Use the same headings as your first list and put it away. Again in about a week get out both lists and review them.

By making these two lists you are taking concrete action. This action may very well help you to organize your thoughts and emotions, and help to put some order/reality into perspective. Once you decide, whatever your decision is, I can assure you that you will feel an immense sense of relief. Once you have made your decision, you can set goals and make a plan of action. This will surely provide you with a sense of direction. Once you make your decision, don't question it too much. Don't let any family member try to intimidate you into feeling guilty or irresponsible for the decision you made. The people who usually pull this trick are the very ones that were never around to help you when you needed them! Believe me, they won't be there in the future to help you, no matter what your decision is!

In the final analysis, life must go on — because it does go on, with or without you. Hopefully life will go on with you whether it is in familiar or unfamiliar patterns. Whenever possible — at least every day — laugh at yourself, with yourself and others. Say positive, helpful, and hopeful things. Be encouraging and encourage others. Say your prayers when you go to bed at night. Don't be afraid or embarrassed to say you are sorry — that you lost your temper, your patience. Before you go to bed tonight, tell someone that you love and care about them. Tell yourself that you did the very best that you could have done today, and that no matter what, you could not have changed the entire course of life's events as much as you would have wished that you could have. Each day do something for yourself, no matter how small it may be — your soul depends on it. Whatever your circumstances may be, deal with them as best as you know how.

So, my family and friends, keep well. Strive to be happy, for surely it will be the lifeline to a positive future for you.

2

The Caregiver's Story

I became a caregiver by default — no one else was in a position to care for my father. I had absolutely no experience in tending to anyone who was ill. My children had the usual childhood diseases, colds and flu, but those things were taken in stride as part of a mother's job. Now I had to care for an elderly man with Parkinson's disease and arteriosclerosis.

My father was a tall, handsome man who, until he was 80 years old, did all his own housework, put his storm windows up in the fall and down in the spring and shoveled his own and most of the neighbors' sidewalks in the worst of Buffalo snowstorms. But at 81 he started failing, his hands started shaking, and he became quite forgetful. Only his pride kept him from seeing a doctor until my brother practically dragged him in for tests. His diseases were those of old age, but once they took hold, they progressed rapidly. Soon it was apparent he could not live alone in our big old family home in the University section.

So I, being the only one single in the family, moved in and became a caregiver, a job that in one way was the most difficult I had ever had, but in another way, one of the most rewarding and educational. Ah, yes, definitely educational.

I am the youngest of seven children. Two of my three brothers are dead, one in a car accident at eight years of age and one at 24 as a pilot in World War II. Therefore, one evening shortly after I had moved into my father's home, my brother, three sisters, and I got together to discuss how my father's care would be handled.

Even though everything didn't happen as we planned it that night, I would suggest that this would be a good starting point for any family in this situation. My brother got a power of attorney from our lawyer and took over the finances. I was given an allowance for keeping the house. I was not working but I had money in the bank to use for my personal needs. Dad would stay in his upstairs room because he was still negotiating the stairs very well — it had a good sturdy bannister on the stairway, the kind they built back in the "old days." The main problem was that Dad would not take his medicine – he either didn't remember or he was just being stubborn. So one of my duties was to give him his medicine. He took two kinds, the one by spoon I put directly into his mouth; the one in pill form I gave him with his water and stood there to make sure he swallowed it every time. It worked – he took his medicine from then on.

One of the most difficult things to face in this situation was caring for the father who had cared so many years for me. He was a wonderful father and I was his baby — a fact which he always made clear to everyone at family gatherings like weddings and funerals, even when I was a mother and grandmother! He had been the kind of father who sang us songs every night after dinner, made us oatmeal in the cold weather, took us for long walks and happy vacations. He had been the head of a large, happy family and now he couldn't remember our names most of the time.

One of Dad's favorite recreations was walking. He loved to walk and he taught all of us to love it, too. At first I let him take his usual walk down to the stores on Bailey Avenue where he'd go into the coffee shop and talk to some of the retired men he knew. He'd go to the bank, to church for a visit, to my brother's or sister's house a few blocks from home. But soon this had to stop. He became very disoriented and a couple of times was really lost and neighbors would call for me to pick him up. I went with him every day for a while, or my son or niece or nephew did, but when he started to "list" from his Parkinson's, his walks had to stop. He was confused and didn't know why, and I felt terrible

having to stop him. Of course, if I had known who to talk to
about it, I might have had him use a walker at that stage, but
I had no idea something like that was available. Eventually I
learned many things were available, but at that stage I was just
blundering through it all.

There were some hurtful times that even now are hard to
think about, much less write about. As my father deteriorated,
his disposition was not always that of the father I remembered.
He would shout at me and criticize me — especially my cooking.
My father had always had a delicate stomach and my mother
had catered to him. Even when we were all small — there is only
ten years difference between me and my oldest sister — she
made Dad separate meals and fussed over each thing he ate. My
mother had died ten years before I had come to stay with my
father, and in the interim he, who had never cooked except that
oatmeal on a winter's morning, started to cook for himself. He
mixed up the most awful concoctions — my mother would have
turned over in her grave if she had seen them. The only time he
ate well was when he went out to eat or ate at one of our houses.

So when I came to take care of him I tried to cook the way
my mother had done. I made him nice fussy meals with just
small portions of everything the way he had always liked. Well,
he didn't care much for my cooking and told me so loudly and
often. He would tell me what a good cook my mother was, and
my sisters and sister-in-law could really cook, not the "slop" I
cooked. I was hurt but put it down to his illness and just kept
plugging along. He'd usually eat — even my cooking — but
sometimes he thought he had just eaten, he couldn't remember.

The hardest thing I had to do came next. I would help Dad
get ready for bed, give him his final medication for the night
(which usually helped him sleep) and then go to my room (on the
same floor) and get some needed rest or read a book to get my
mind back on track. Well, Dad got to getting up in the middle of
the night. He would get completely dressed for outdoors, even
his hat, and I, by that time sleeping, wasn't even aware of it until
one night when they called me from a little restaurant at Bailey
and Broadway where Dad had gone in his working days. Dad
had come in there, they all knew him, he talked coherently for

a while and then got all confused and didn't know where he was or how to get home. He had gone there on the bus, and I didn't know where he had gotten the money, but he did it. Well, from then on I had to lock the front door at night and keep the key with me.

That stopped Dad's nocturnal wandering, but he still got up every night, hammered on my door, screaming for me to get the key and let him out. It was heart-breaking. So I'd get up and there he'd be all dressed for work, he insisted he had to get to work. We'd spend the rest of the night talking (Dad would talk, I would listen) about the people at work. He would go on and on and sometimes he'd call me by my mother's name thinking he had come home from work and was telling her his day. This went on for a long time. I just gave up sleeping unless I was sure he was definitely sleeping during the day.

His Parkinson's was getting worse and he was shaking terribly. I helped him to eat and dress, but he was needing more care all the time. I was beginning to wear down.

You might wonder at this point, where was my family? Well, that's a good question. They came a few times in the beginning when I was just settling in, and they continued with the financial aspects, but usually I was alone with Dad twenty-four hours a day. The family never relieved me or said they would stay with him while I went shopping or to church or to my daughter's. When they saw I was coping they let me cope. They all had excuses why they couldn't take him. No room, kids too noisy, husband wouldn't like it, etc., etc. My one sister took him and was going to keep him all afternoon and for dinner. She had him back home in an hour. The same with my older sister. My brother did come to visit. My brother usually complained that I wasn't feeding him right or had some other criticism. I think my father told him I was mean to him. This was not my father, it was the illness, I realized, but it still hurt.

Now, when I look back, I realize and I would tell this to other people in these circumstances, that we should have had a schedule made and though I would be the full time caregiver, they would have to take turns also.

Who did help — and I would like to share this as something to think about if you ever need to: grandchildren (some of them) were wonderful with their grandfather. Three of them in particular — my oldest son, my nephew, and niece-in-law — all had a fabulous rapport with my father. My son would listen to Dad's meanderings, and take him for rides in his van (which was quite comfortable for Dad). My nephew went out in the yard and threw a baseball back and forth with my father and Dad loved it. He had been quite a baseball player in his day. My niece was studying physical therapy and she used some of the techniques she was learning on my father and they had good results. He seemed to love being with the young people and was quite alert when they came around. I will always be grateful to them.

One of my unlovely characteristics has always been my pride. Stubbornness isn't far behind either. I needed help, badly, but I didn't know where to turn and was too proud and too stubborn to do something about it. So I just kept muddling through, lacking sleep, finding my father needing more and more care. Plus keeping the large house was different from taking care of my small apartment. I needed to get out once in a while and my father needed to get out as well.

Well, the answer came when an old acquaintance called — a young lady who was working on her doctorate in social work. I told her just what was happening and the need for some kind of help. She directed me to Social Services. What a godsend! A gentleman from Social Services came over and interviewed me and my father. He told me the things that were available for us. What I finally opted for was an aide to come in one day a week and care for Dad while I took some free time for myself. The other thing we decided to try was to get Dad out of the house occasionally. There was a program for elderly people like him who were not well, but ambulatory. One day a week a bus picked him up and he was taken to a center where they worked on crafts (if they were able) or just talked or sang — counselors talked one on one with the oldsters. It worked. Dad seemed to like it and even though he couldn't participate in crafts, he liked the music and became more alert just from the attention and getting away from home.

Things went on like this for a while but then other problems cropped up. During his checkup, Dad was found to have some problems with his colon. He went into the hospital for tests. He had colon cancer. He started failing, he became more frail. When one night he fell down the stairs I realized that other arrangements would need to be made. My brother and sisters and I got together with the doctor and we put Dad in the Veteran's Hospital. We decided we did not want any operations, as his cancer had metastasized, but just keep him as free of pain as possible. He never came home again.

I stayed at the house, hoping maybe by some miracle he'd return, but when he didn't, I started getting things together. I visited him often at the hospital and so did my brother and sisters. When my son graduated from college in Oklahoma, my other son, my daughter and I flew to the ceremonies, and the day before we returned, my father died. I was sorry I could not be with him, but I was glad his suffering was over.

My job as caregiver was over, but after the funeral there were still the house and furnishings to be taken care of, and I needed to find a job and a place to live. My brother and one of my sisters were being very nasty and even though Dad have left everything he owned equally to the five of us, there were terrible hard feelings. I had heard that families had all kinds of disagreements during these times, but I never thought it would happen to my family. It did. My sister didn't speak to me for a year over absolutely nothing, but all is now resolved and we are friends again. By the way, none of them ever said "Thank you."

I said in the beginning of this article that it was a difficult job but a rewarding one, and that is very true. I would not give up those months with my father for anything on earth. I, who thought she couldn't do anything as difficult as caring for a sick, elderly person, did it. I told my father often what a wonderful dad he had been and how much I loved him. I never would have been able to do that under ordinary circumstances. Those things tend not to be said in life's day-to-day circumstances, so I was glad I had a chance. And even though Dad was confused and sometimes not very nice to me, I feel he knew I was doing the best I could. I'm sure that, even for him, it was hard to have your daughter take care of you. He had pride, too — where do you think I got it from?

What did I learn? Not to be so darn independent and stubborn. Ask for help. After I learned about Social Services everything was much easier. I wish I had dealt better with my brother and sisters. Regular conferences would have been a good idea. Communication was not good and that caused many problems.

I hope some of what I have written will help you understand one person's caregiver situation.

3

Hospital Discharge Planning

Introduction

You've made the decision to return home after a tiresome hospital stay. Who do you turn to for help to smoothly and skillfully assist you to return to these familiar surroundings? The hospital discharge planner.

According to the American Hospital Association, discharge planning is a coordinated program established by a health care institution ensuring that each patient will be provided with a planned program for continued services and follow-up mechanisms.

Discharge planners are generally nurses or social workers who coordinate this safe movement of a patient from hospital to home while preserving continuity of care. The discharge planner prepares for every patient's discharge by first making a comprehensive assessment which culminates in the development of an individualized care plan for each patient and their significant others.

Although a patient's discharge occurs at the end of his or her hospital stay, discharge planning occurs the minute a patient enters the hospital.

Discharge Planners — What They Do
and What You Can Expect

Upon admission to many hospitals, each patient and their significant others are given a patient information guide booklet. Tucked away in this booklet, among information on policies and procedures, is information concerning a patient's hospital discharge. Imagine! The day a person enters a hospital is the day that they are expected to think about when they will leave! Such terms as: certified home health agency, long-term home health care program, hospice care, nursing and other community services, counseling and support services, financial assistance and legal services, and durable medical equipment may be mentioned almost immediately.

Once a discharge planning nurse becomes involved in the patient's plan of care, he or she coordinates the post-hospital plan for that patient. The discharge planner meets with the patient and their significant others to determine the patient's needs upon discharge. The patient's doctor, primary nurse, therapists (physical therapist and occupational therapist), nutritionist, medical social worker, and all others integral to the patient are consulted.

When meeting with the discharge planner, it is important that openness and honesty are apparent in order to establish an effective post-hospital care plan. Remember, discharge planners are your advocates. They are there to assist you in setting up the best home care plan — one that works for you!

The discharge planner will explain what assistance is available and what is unavailable under your individual insurance. In order for home care to be covered under insurance, there must be a need for skilled nursing (something that only a registered nurse is qualified to do). However, these regulations vary from state to state, and from county to county. Even though a patient may need help with bathing, eating, or walking, these activities are considered to be custodial, and are thus not covered under insurance. If these services are needed, the discharge planner can assist in making the appropriate arrangements through private agencies.

If finances are limited and the patient is eligible for public assistance, the discharge planner will assist in obtaining this as well.

The discharge planner can ease the anxieties regarding the transition from hospital to home by arranging for home care under the patient's insurance if possible. The planner also can arrange for the caregiver to come into the hospital for education regarding transferring a patient, feeding, bathing, and bedmaking. The discharge planner also assists in obtaining needed equipment.

The discharge planner can assist caregivers in finding local groups (clusters) or synagogue or church organizations that may be able to provide support and/or actual assistance with patient care. Discharge planners can also assist in finding respite care. This is necessary so that the caregiver receives the proper rest so they can continue to care for their loved one.

In essence, the efficient and yet personal transition from hospital to home occurs because of discharge planners who care and want to see the best post-hospital plan for their patient and patient's caregivers.

Questions for Your Discharge Planner

1. What kinds of services do I need?

2. Can I make some of my own decisions regarding kinds of services I need?

3. How will I pay for the services I need?

4. Can I decide who will provide me with the services I need?

5. What equipment will I need at home? How do I obtain it?

6. Are most agencies licensed, bonded, and insured? How do I find out?

7. Are all home care employees specially trained? Are they supervised? (If so, by who and how?)

8. Do I have a voice in my own home care plan?

9. Is the agency's staff available to me 24 hours a day? How can I contact them when I need to?

10. Does the agency keep my private doctor informed?

To the average person coming into a hospital, the discharge planner is probably the least known of all health care professionals. The average person also does not always know what services are available to them when they return home. As early as possible, after your admission, ask to speak personally to your discharge planner. He or she can put your mind at ease, which will surely speed your recovery.

4

Preparing Your Home for a Person with a Disability

A person's home is, essentially, an extension of their personality. We all dream of one day owning "a place of our own." In fact, a house is probably the single largest investment that most of us will ever make in our lifetime. When buying or renting, we consider many factors: cost, location, and aesthetics, to name a few. Rarely, however, do we ever stop to consider that due to an accident, illness, or even the normal process of aging, one's "dream house" can become a nightmare. The dwelling that we worked our entire lives to afford can become our greatest enemy. It has been said that "a man's home is his castle"; however, that castle may ultimately become a prison, and its occupants, prisoners; prisoners in their own home.

When one becomes disabled, for whatever reason, many of the features of the house which were previously taken for granted, can combine to make life difficult, not only for the disabled individual, but for their caregiver as well. This chapter will explore some of the most common trouble areas in the house, and describe methods to make life a little easier and safer, for its occupants.

Access In and Around the House

When arriving home from the hospital, the first problem that many people encounter is that of access into and out of the house, as well as to different rooms within it. When normal walking, or ambulation, is no longer possible, and one must be assisted by a cane, walker, or wheelchair, one may find that it is difficult and often impossible to get into the house and move about from room to room. Even more distressing, once inside the house, they are unable to easily exit. This, essentially, makes that person a prisoner who must spend what may seem like an eternity, in their home; unable to fully enjoy those activities available in the outside community and beyond. What is worse is that in case of an emergency, escape from the house may often be impossible. It is essential that access to the home be accommodated to the disabled individual.

Ramps

Because most houses do not have direct access to ground level and are accessible only by steps, many homes require the addition of ramps to allow individuals in wheelchairs, and those with walkers and canes, to enter and exit more easily. Many people often build their own ramps to remedy this situation. Unfortunately, these ramps are frequently constructed improperly, and can be dangerous to the user. Therefore, certain guidelines should be followed when building a ramp, or having one built by friends, family members, or even professionals.

Before beginning any ramp system, review all of the entrances to your home and consider the following: Which door is the widest? Which has the fewest steps? Which has the best/most efficient overall access?

Probably the most common error in ramp construction is that of improper slope or pitch. People will often construct a makeshift ramp by placing a long board over the existing steps, with a resulting slope which is much too steep to be negotiated safely (Fig. 1).

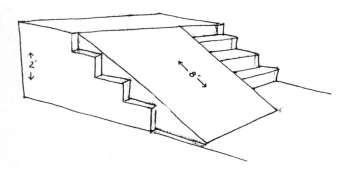

Fig. 1   Improper ramp on stairway.

It is recommended that the length of the ramp be determined by the following formula: for every inch of rise, there should be twelve inches of ramp. To construct a ramp for a two foot high front porch, for example, one would require one foot of ramp to each of twenty-four inches of rise (1' x 24" = 24'), or twenty-four feet of ramp (Fig. 2). Although this requires more building material, it makes it easier for the disabled person to negotiate the ramp, or if the person is being pushed in a wheelchair, it makes it easier for the attendant.

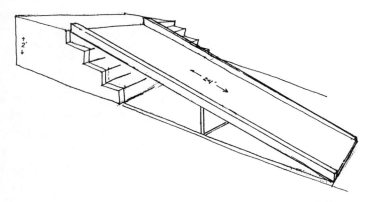

Fig. 2   Proper ramp slope for stairway.

A long ramp can often be impractical due to space considerations, as well as the individual's endurance level. In these cases it is advisable to change the direction of the ramp at equal intervals by installing landings. These landings will also provide rest stops, if needed. The landings should be large enough to allow a wheelchair to turn easily; they are usually four feet square (Fig. 3).

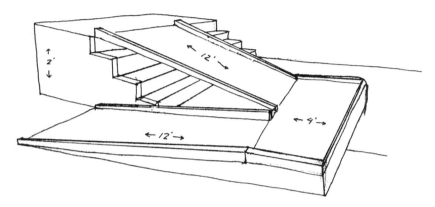

Fig. 3   Proper ramp slope for stairway using alternate directions.

The ramp should always include a side railing to prevent accidental falls, and should be covered with a non-skid material to prevent slipping. Bare plywood, as well as indoor/outdoor carpeting, can be extremely slippery when wet and should not be used. Special textured paints or Dycem are safer. Footholds, placed at equal intervals, are also recommended. However, they must not be as wide, or wider than the wheels of a wheelchair, as they would interfere with its propulsion.

Many people prefer not to have, or cannot have, a permanent ramp installed at their place of residence. In these instances, a portable, collapsible aluminum ramp can be employed. This ramp can be installed and removed in a matter of minutes, and laid over the top of the existing steps. Because the pitch of the ramp would be too steep to negotiate safely, the process can be made easier and safer by using an electric winch, which is secured at the top of the landing. The winch has forward and reverse capabilities, and can lower and raise a person in a wheelchair. The wheelchair must always face towards the top of the stairs to prevent its occupant from pitching forward, out of the chair. A seatbelt should always be used during the transport. With the winch cable securely fastened to the wheelchair cross members, the person can be safely raised or lowered on the ramp at a comfortable speed (Fig. 4) (See reference at end of chapter).

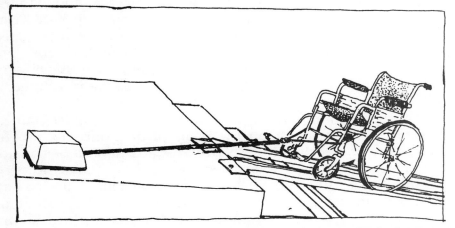

Fig. 4   Ramp and winch system.

One final option is a wheelchair lift. This allows the wheelchair to be safely and easily transported from ground to upper levels and vice versa. However, these lifts are very expensive and may not be covered by insurance.

Doorways

When one becomes disabled, particularly when one must use a wheelchair, doorways can become a source of difficulty and inaccessibility. Many doorways, especially bathroom doors, are not designed to accommodate wheelchairs, and frequently bar access to the wheelchair bound. The average doorway is twenty-eight inches wide before the trim is added; bathroom doors are typically narrower. The standard adult wheelchair, on the other hand, is 25 1/2" wide. This makes access difficult, at best, and dangerous or impossible, at worst. However, there are some modifications which can be made, which will allow easier access.

The most logical solution, of course, is to widen the existing doorways. Unfortunately, most of us cannot afford this option. Therefore, other alternatives must be chosen.

Perhaps the easiest modification is to remove the door from the hinges. When the door is removed, the doorway can be increased by up to 2 1/2 valuable inches. A curtain can be installed to protect one's privacy. By also removing the inner molding of the door jamb, another one inch can be added to the entryway. If it is not feasible to remove the door, special hinges can be purchased which compensate for some of the space used by the door by allowing it to swing further away from the door frame than a conventional hinge. Finally, by removing or modifying the doorsill, access can be more easily facilitated.

Another option, if an individual must use a wheelchair, is to select the wheelchair on the basis of its utility within the home. Narrow wheelchairs are available and should be considered if accessibility is a problem. A professional should be consulted regarding the selection of a wheelchair, as it is an extremely important piece of equipment, and should not be randomly selected (refer to Chapter 5 on Durable Medical Equipment).

Stairways

Stairways can present major obstacles within the home, regardless of whether one uses a wheelchair, a walker, or a cane. Other medical problems such as cardiac or pulmonary conditions may also make it difficult to utilize stairways. A fall down the stairs can result in serious injury. Therefore, attention should be given to this area.

Those individuals who are ambulatory, with or without assistance, will find that the task is made easier by using handrails. These should be professionally installed on all stairways and should be sturdy enough to support a person's full body weight if necessary. Handrails should be installed on both sides of the stairs in order to accommodate the person's dominant hand or, in the case of a stroke, their stronger side, while going up or down the stairs. Foreign objects should never be left on the stairs or the landings, as these can cause one to trip and fall. Non-slip material should be installed on wooden or linoleum stairs. For persons with poor eyesight it is often useful to paint the edge of each step with a bright color to reduce the possibility of missing a step and falling. In all cases, stairways should be well lit to prevent misplaced footing and resulting falls.

For the individual who is confined to a wheelchair, the story is a bit different. A ramp is not a viable alternative as the slope would be impossible to negotiate. Unless an individual is fortunate enough to have an elevator in their home, the upstairs of the house is, most likely, off limits. If the bedroom and bathroom facilities are located upstairs, you may want to consider moving the person's living quarters to the ground floor. If no downstairs toilet is available, a commode can be used instead. Although this scenario may not be the most preferable, it does have some advantages. First, it saves a great deal of exertion on the part of the person and the caregiver, allowing more energy to be used for activities which both parties may enjoy. Second, by being closer to the outside doorways, the person is allowed faster, easier, and safer escape in the event of a medical emergency or fire. Finally, the person is closer to "the action" within the home, rather than being confined to "the sickroom."

Stairlifts can allow wheelchair bound individuals and people with arthritis, Multiple Sclerosis, Amyotrophic Lateral Sclerosis (Lou Gerhig's Disease), Alzheimer's Disease, or cardiac conditions, to achieve safe access, both up and down stairs. Unfortunately, these are expensive items, and may not be available to many individuals through their insurance.

General Guidelines for Access within the Home

There are many things which we take for granted as able bodied individuals. However, when one becomes disabled, many of these little things can become nuisances or even sources of danger. Below are listed some of the more common problems faced by the newly disabled individual.

Carpeting is a luxury which many people have in their homes. However, if one has a reduced ability to ambulate, or must depend on a wheelchair to get around, carpeting can become an obstacle to independence. Although we are not recommending that carpeting be removed, the drawbacks should be mentioned. Generally, the thicker the pile of the carpet, the more difficult it is to walk or roll a wheelchair on. Shag and plush carpets are the most difficult, while the indoor/outdoor and commercial types are the easiest. The thickness of the carpet padding will also affect mobility. Often these obstacles can be overcome by using a lightweight wheelchair or one with pneumatic (air filled) tires, instead of those made of solid rubber. Wooden, tile, or linoleum floor surfaces are easiest to negotiate. However, they have their own problems as they are more conducive to slips and falls due to spilled liquids and/or highly waxed surfaces. Throw rugs can also be dangerous if one trips over an edge and therefore, these should be used with caution. If throw rugs are used they should be secured with double faced tape or an equivalent fastener and are not recommended on stairs or landings. We recommend, however, that throw rugs be removed altogether.

The house in general, should be free from clutter, particularly in high traffic areas. Electrical and telephone cords should be placed out of the way to prevent accidental falls. Cords should never be placed near doorways or stairs.

Pets are often an important part of peoples lives, but they can also be a source of danger to a disabled individual. Pet owners should be careful that pets are not underfoot while the disabled individual is walking about.

Chair and Sofa Adaptations

It is often difficult for many persons to get into and out of a favorite chair or sofa. Most furniture is not designed for the disabled. Many people frequently end up spending the majority of their "up" time sitting in a wheelchair, because it is too difficult and/or painful to get in and out of a favorite chair. This is unfortunate. However, it is an easy situation to remedy. By placing the chair or sofa on a raised platform (Fig. 5), the disabled individual is placed in a position to sit down and stand up more easily. If the person requires assistance with their transfers, a higher surface also makes it easier for the caregiver, and may prevent lower back injuries. A platform of this type can be easily constructed from a piece of one inch plywood cut slightly wider than the base of the chair. Two-by-fours can then be attached to the underside of the plywood to provide the needed height. It is important to note that when raising the furniture height, the platform should be constructed in such a way as to prevent the legs of the furniture from sliding off; such as by placing a raised border around the edge of the platform, for example. Commercial leg risers, which attach to the existing chair legs, can also be purchased to increase the height of the chair.

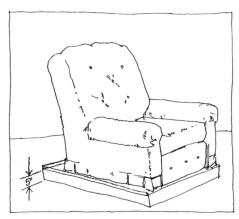

Fig. 5   Raised platform for armchair.

Depending on their medical diagnoses, many people who have trouble standing may be eligible for electric lift armchairs. These are very useful and can be extremely helpful to these individuals and their caregivers, as well. One needs to consult a durable medical equipment supplier to find out if they are eligible for these chairs. (see Chapter 5, page 61)

Devices for Easy Living

We are fortunate to live in an era of readily available technology. Many commercially available devices can make life easier for everyone – especially for the disabled homebound individual. Environmental control systems can allow an individual to control virtually every electric device from anywhere in the house. Devices such as electric garage door openers, electric can openers, table top stoves, and microwave ovens can foster safety and independence, and should be considered for use if possible.

Cordless telephones are another relatively new innovation which can allow an individual immediate access to a telephone for whatever reason. Cordless phones can be carried in a holster or in a wheelchair for easy access and convenience. Aside from their immeasurable usefulness in emergencies, they reduce the need to "run" to a stationary telephone, and eliminate unnecessary and dangerous telephone cords stretching across a room. Many models feature an auto-dialer feature which can be useful, especially in emergencies.

If a person lives alone, or is alone for long periods of time, a personal emergency response system should be considered. This system provides the individual with the ability to contact emergency assistance by pressing a button on a unit which can be worn around the wrist or neck. There are many providers of this type of service throughout the country. Before choosing a given firm, the reliability of the firm should be investigated to ensure that help will arrive when summoned.

Considerations for Specific Rooms

Although many of us live in houses with a number of different rooms, there are certain rooms which are common to most houses: the bedroom, the bathroom, and the kitchen. As these will be the rooms that many people will be concerned with following a disability, we shall discuss these three rooms in some detail.

The Bedroom

When recovering from a disability, at least initially, it is probable that an individual will spend a great deal of time in the bedroom. It is, therefore, essential that this room be arranged in such a way as to promote safety, ease of transfers, and utility. As already stated, if the bedroom is located upstairs, and is essentially inaccessible, you might consider relocating the bedroom to the downstairs.

The overall size of the room should be evaluated and furniture rearranged if necessary, to allow for wheelchair access and maneuverability, transfer ease, and safety. Again, all unnecessary clutter should be removed from the traffic areas and all cords should be out of the way.

The bed should be situated in such a way as to allow for easy access and safe transfers, both in and out of the bed. Ideally, the bed should be accessible from both sides in order to better facilitate transfers (see Chapter 7 for transfer techniques) and care of the person (Chapter 6). For example, if the person has had a stroke, access into and out of the bed should be toward their stronger side, which requires access from both sides of the bed.

If the individual will be using their own bed, it is important that the mattress be firm to assist in bed mobility. If the mattress is too soft, a board can be inserted between the mattress and the boxspring, for additional firmness. Full wave waterbeds are difficult to maneuver in and are not recommended for someone who has difficulty with bed mobility.

People often require or request a hospital bed following hospitalization. Although hospital beds may reinforce the sick role, they do have their advantages; particularly in positioning and transferring the person, as well as reducing edema and accumulation of fluid in the lungs. Hospital beds are available in manual, semi-electric, and fully electric types. It is best to consult your therapist or durable medical equipment supplier prior to buying or renting such a bed.

People sometimes have trouble sitting up or pulling themselves up in bed. When this is a problem, an overhead trapeze bar can help facilitate the process by allowing the person to pull themselves up in bed. Trapeze bars come in two different styles: headboard mounted and free standing. The headboard style is recommended only if the headboard is made of steel, such as a hospital bed. The free standing model sits on the floor, behind and under the bed, and eliminates the need for a steel headboard. However, they are not as firmly anchored as the attached unit. Both types are available with a swivel feature which allows the trapeze to move from one side to another, thereby increasing the ease of transfers. We recommend the swivel version for this reason.

People who spend a great deal of time in bed may become uncomfortable and are prone to bedsores (decubiti). For these individuals, special mattresses may be indicated to reduce or prevent these problems. The popular egg-crate-type pads, which are frequently used by many people, may not be sufficient for an individual who spends a great deal of time in bed. Although they are inexpensive, they do not reduce the possibility of bedsores during prolonged bedrest – particularly if the individual is extremely thin, or has a condition such as diabetes which may compromise skin integrity. In cases such as these there are other alternatives. **Consult with your physician before you obtain any mattress.**

Flotation mattresses, filled with water or gel, can help the person to shift their body weight easily, thus reducing the possibility of bed sores. They are extremely comfortable and maintain a constant room temperature. These mattresses are approximately one and a half inches thick when filled and are easy to install by simply placing them on top of the existing mattresses. A full size twin bed model costs less than $100.

Alternating air mattresses have two separate air bladders which inflate and deflate, on alternating cycles, and shift the person's body weight from one area to another, preventing constant pressure on any area which comes into contact with the bed, and assisting in preventing bedsores. The pressure is controlled by an extremely quiet air pump and the shift is so subtle as to be imperceptible to the person. Alternating air mattresses can be purchased or rented.

If the person has difficulty walking, or if the bathroom is too far away from the bedroom, a commode should be placed next to the bed. This will allow the person to merely stand and pivot, in order to transfer from the bed to the commode.

Arrange closets and dressers to allow easy access to belongings. It is often useful to lower the closet rod to allow the person to reach clothing without having to ask for assistance.

The Bathroom

The bathroom is, undoubtedly, the most frequently used room in any household. It is also the most dangerous, and most household accidents occur in this room. When one becomes incapacitated, the chances of an accident in the bathroom increase substantially. It is therefore essential that this room be given special consideration when attempting to accommodate a disabled loved one.

As a rule, bathrooms are typically small, with little room to navigate a wheelchair or, in many instances, even a walker. As already mentioned, the doorway is usually narrower than others in the house, and access can be difficult, at best. If a wheelchair is necessary, a narrow or travel model should be considered.

Toilet adaptations

Toilets are not designed with disabilities in mind, and are typically too low for many people to get on and off easily. Fortunately, there are many ways to make this easier.

For the individual who has minor difficulty sitting down on, or standing up from the toilet, commercially available grab bars can assist in these motions (Fig. 6). Grab bars should be professionally installed, with the screws securely anchored in wall studs, to prevent them from pulling out of the wall under a person's body weight. Toilet paper holders and towel bars should never be used as a substitute for a grab bar! They are not designed to withstand great pressures and will break or separate from the wall, possibly causing severe injury.

Another option to consider is the installation of toilet assist rails (Fig. 7). These are height adjustable units which attach directly to the toilet, eliminating the need for drilling into walls. The toilet assist rails give the toilet an armchair effect and allow the individual to push with their arms, making toilet transfers easier and safer.

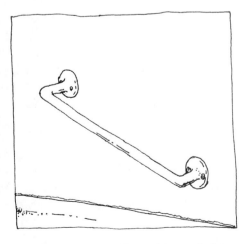

Fig. 6   Wall mount grab bar.

The height of the toilet seat can be increased by the installation of a commercially a-vailable raised toilet seat. These seats place the person at a mechanical advantage which is more conducive to standing or sitting. They are secured to the existing toilet, and can be removed and reinstalled quickly and easily. We recommend the type with the anti-tip feature for added safety and security.

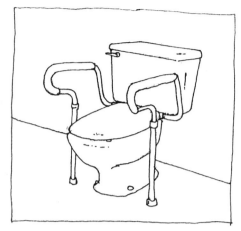

Fig. 7   Toilet assist rails.

By removing its plastic bucket, many commode seats, such as the 'three-in-one' commode, can be placed over the toilet and act as a raised toilet seat. The bucket can be replaced by a splash guard, which is similar to a bucket, but without a bottom. The commode seat offers an increased height advantage, as well as the support of side arms for ease in standing and sitting. It has a further advantage in that Medicare/Medicaid will pay for a commode, while they will not pay for a raised toilet seat.

Bathtub/Shower Adaptations

Perhaps one of the greatest disappointments to a newly disabled individual is the inability to take a bath or shower due to the inaccessibility of the bathtub. Many persons are unable to transfer into or out of the tub easily or safely and therefore must settle for a less than refreshing sponge bath. The unfortunate reality, however, is that many of these individuals are not aware that there are many adaptations which can facilitate safe and easy bathtub transfers.

For the individual with generalized weakness, decreased balance or range of motion (ROM), perhaps the easiest adaptation is the installation of grab bars. As previously mentioned, these should be installed professionally, and the person and/or caregiver should consult an occupational therapist for the proper location and angle of the bar. Again, towel racks or soap dishes should never be used as a substitute for a grab bar. Tub mount grab bars (Fig. 8) can also be used to allow safe, easy access into and out of the tub. These are commercially available and can be installed and removed quickly and easily. These bars clamp to the side of the tub and will not damage the porcelain. If the tub is equipped with sliding glass doors, these should be removed and replaced with a shower curtain. These doors interfere with bathtub transfers and can make transfers more difficult and dangerous.

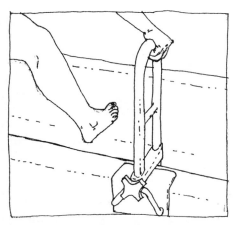

Fig. 8   Tub mount grab bar.

For added safety, the bathtub should always have a non-skid mat or strips to prevent falls. The mats are easy to remove and clean and will not damage the tub. The strips are fastened by adhesive and are more or less permanent. Many modern tubs and shower stalls are equipped with textured, non-slip surfaces which also work well. A rubber based bathmat should also be used on the outside of the tub. This will prevent the person from slipping on the bathroom floor after transferring out of the tub.

Bathbenches

Many individuals find that they cannot sit down in the tub, even with the assistance of grab bars. For these individuals, a bathtub seat or bath transfer bench are often an easy solution. These adjustable seats are available in a variety of styles to meet any individual's special needs (Figs. 9-11). Although they are commercially available, an occupational thera-

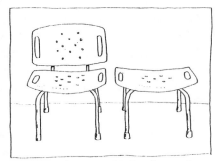

Fig. 9   Bathtub seats.

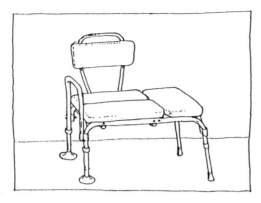

**Fig. 10   Freestanding bathtub
              transfer bench.**

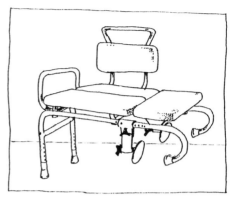

**Fig. 11   Clamp on bathtub
              transfer bench.**

pist should be consulted before one is purchased. The wrong
bathtub seat can be not just a waste of money – it can also be
dangerous.

The major disadvantage of many tubseats is that they do
not allow the bather to get all the way down into the tub. This
is not a problem if one is content to take a shower only. However,
many people do not like showers or prefer to soak in a nice, hot
bath. For these persons, a hydraulic tub seat is a convenient
alternative (Fig. 12). These are also commercially available and
come in a number of different styles. These seats are connected
to the showerhead or faucet, and are raised and lowered by
filling and emptying pistons or
water bladders, thus allowing
the bather to get up and down
in the tub without having to
stand. These are generally more
expensive than standard tubseats (from $400 to $1000) and
are usually not covered by insurance. However, many people
find them to be worth the expense.

For the individual who is
confined to bed and cannot be

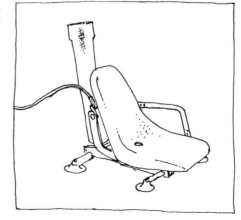

Fig. 12   Hydraulic bath bench.

safely or easily transferred into the tub or shower stall, there are a number of inflatable bed bathtubs, which are relatively easy for the caregiver to install and bathe the person. Furthermore, shampoo basins can allow an individual to have their hair and scalp thoroughly cleaned while laying in bed or sitting in a chair.

Shower Stall Adaptations

Shower stalls are generally easier to get into and out of. However, there are some adaptations which should be considered.

Again, a non-slip mat should always be used in the shower stall. A hole may need to be cut into the mat, to allow for proper drainage, however, and adhesive strips may be more practical in this situation. Grab bars should also be installed to prevent slips and falls. A tub or shower seat is essential for an individual with generalized weakness, poor endurance, or balance.

A hand held shower head is a convenient item which allows an individual to thoroughly cleanse his or her body. These can be purchased in a variety of commercial and DME stores, and are easily installed in either a shower stall or bathtub. Some types have an on/off switch on the showerhead, which eliminates the need to reach to the stationary water faucet. Other models can be mounted on a vertical bar which allows adjustable stationary placement, if so desired.

The biggest concern in the bathroom is that of safety. Many of these adaptations can also be useful to those individuals who may not be disabled, but find that, due to increasing age and loss of physical function, bathing and toileting is becoming increasingly more difficult.

The Kitchen

For many people, homemakers in particular, once they are incapacitated, the kitchen is rarely, if ever, used again. Many people become overwhelmed at the prospect of attempting to function in a room which is not designed to meet the needs of a disabled cook.

The primary consideration for the disabled homemaker is the general layout of the kitchen. Although there is little that can be done to rearrange major appliances, such as the stove and refrigerator, there are many other changes and adaptations which can help to make meal preparation and clean up safer and easier. The kitchen should be ergonomically designed, that is, it should be arranged in such a way as to save as much work as possible, to make tasks easier and safer.

The modern kitchen frequently contains many labor saving devices which can greatly assist in meal preparation. Items such as electric can openers, food processors, microwave ovens, and dishwashers can make life a great deal easier for the general population. For the disabled homemaker, however, they can also mean the difference between making meals or depending on others to do so. As convenient as these appliances may be, there are other considerations that must be kept in mind in order to promote safe independence in the kitchen.

For many, especially those in wheelchairs, kitchen cabinets are frequently too high, and many items cannot be easily or safely reached. Therefore, these should be evaluated and rearranged according to the following guidelines:

1) Items which are frequently used, such as spices, pots and pans, dishes, etc., as well as heavy items such as crockpots, cans or jars, etc., should be stored in lower cabinets, preferably in those below the counter. This will eliminate the need for unnecessary reaching and accidentally dropping items. Lighter items, as well as infrequently used items, can be stored in the higher cabinets, if necessary.

2) Keep as much of the counters and table clear to allow sliding of objects from one place to another. This will eliminate the need to carry items.

3) A wheeled cart can allow one to move heavy and/or multiple objects from one place to another with minimal effort. Some models can be folded up for storage when not in use. For those in wheelchairs, a securely mounted wheelchair lapboard can also be used for this purpose.

Some Common Household Problems and Possible Solutions

The following table lists some common problems which may be encountered by disabled individuals in their home, as well as some possible solutions to these problems.

Note: Most of the adaptive devices suggested in the solutions column can be obtained at durable medical equipment suppliers, through catalogues, or at commercial and specialty stores. These are only suggestions and are by no means the only possibilities to help you to solve some problems that you may encounter.

PROBLEM	SOLUTION
Unable to reach objects on shelves	• Move heavy and frequently used items to lower shelves
Unable to lift heavy objects	• Slide objects instead of lifting • Roll items on skateboard • Transport items on tea/utility cart
Unable to turn lamps on/off	• Replace standard lamp-switch with extra large knobs • Install touch or sound activators for lamps • Use timers for automatic on/off control of lamps • Connect frequently used lamps to wall switches
Difficulty turning control	• Use adapted turning handle
Difficulty turning door knobs	• Install door knob extensions to increase leverage • Replace knobs with pushbar

PROBLEM	SOLUTION
Difficulty manipulating keys in locks	• Attach keys to key turner for extra leverage • Install electronic keypad to operate lock
Unable to see back burners of stoves from wheelchair	• Install a mirror at 45 degree angle over stove
Unable to carry objects while using walker	• Use walker basket/bag/tray • Use heavy-duty utility cart
Unable to carry objects while in wheelchair	• Use wheelchair laptray • Use wheelchair bag/pouch
Difficulty getting on/off toilet	• Use raised toilet seat • Toilet assist rails • Wall mount grab bar(s) • Place commode seat over toilet (replace bucket with splash-guard)
Difficulty getting in/out arm-chair, sofa, etc.	• Raise chair on platform • Leg extenders • Electric lift chair
Difficulty getting in/out of bathtub with decreased safety	• Tub transfer bench • Bath seat • Hydraulic bath seat • Grab bars (tub mount/wall mount) • Non-slip bathmat in tub • Non-slip bath rug outside of tub • Remove sliding glass doors (if present) • Install hand held shower

PROBLEM	SOLUTION
Person is extremely difficult to transfer, causing danger to both person and caregiver	• Hoyer lift or similar hydraulic/electric lift system • Transfer with two or more persons
Objects move around when attempting to perform activities with one hand	• Use Dycem non-slip pad or damp washcloth under object to prevent slipping
Difficulty manipulating scissors due to arthritis or weakness	• Use loop scissors which automatically open when handle is released • Electric scissors
Difficulty opening containers	• There are a number of devices available for this problem: Jar and can openers, tab-grabbers, plastic bag openers, zip-lock bag sealers and pill bottle openers (request non-child proof medication bottles if there are no children around)

Conclusion

Although it is easy to describe the "perfect" design or adaptation for a home, it is not always easy to achieve due to many factors such as money, space, time and effort. This chapter has attempted to present some of the more important considerations for the disabled individual returning home. Many of the problems presented by the environment can be overcome by simple adaptations; but not necessarily all of them. Many of these modifications can make life easier and simpler for not only the person, but for the caregiver as well. Safety and simplicity are the keys for all involved parties. Being ill or disabled is difficult enough, without having to engage in a constant battle with the environment.

Before you make any home modifications or obtain any assistive devices or equipment, we highly recommend that you get a professional evaluation of your needs. Contact a local rehabilitation center or a home health care agency for such an evaluation.

References

Tigges, K.N., Marcil, W.M. (1986). "Maximizing Quality of Life for the Housebound Patient." The American Journal of Hospice Care, 3:1, Jan/Feb. pp. 21-23.

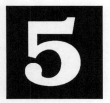

How to Select a Durable Medical Supply Company

You have just been given the responsibility of obtaining medical supply equipment for your spouse, a parent, or perhaps just a good friend that you are trying to help out. If you are like most people, you have never had reason to purchase such equipment, and so have no past experiences to help guide your purchases. Having been a pharmacist and owner of a durable medical equipment and supply company for over 20 years, I would like to share with you some very realistic and practical suggestions.

Selecting the correct equipment initially will eliminate the necessity of making a second purchase of similar equipment in the future. You have a list of needed equipment or supplies, prepared perhaps with the help of a hospital discharge planner, a nurse, a rehabilitation specialist, or a physical or occupational therapist. These professionals can be of tremendous value in suggesting the equipment needed, but the final selection and purchase is up to you. Who do you turn to? The yellow pages of your phone book will give you the names of many suppliers under the "Hospital Medical Supply" section. Friends or relatives who have faced a similar situation may help guide you, and perhaps your own physician will be able to offer advice. It is the practice of hospital discharge planners and physical and occupational therapists to give you a list of the many suppliers in your city, but this is not much better than the yellow pages.

Many professionals will hesitate to recommend just one supplier, but may be willing to suggest several. Hopefully the lists, recommendations and suggestions of suppliers will get you started, and off you go. Set your goal at going to at least two or three suppliers and you will soon begin to see that there is a difference in medical supply companies. If possible, take someone else along with you, such as an adult son or daughter or a good friend who knows you. Whenever possible/feasible, take the patient with you. It will be much easier to make final selections if you have an interested sounding board who has visited and heard the conversations and has seen the equipment with you. I am sure you have been in stores where you felt the salesperson was very helpful and interested in helping you make a selection, and you have been in stores where you felt the salesperson was only interested in taking your money. In purchasing medical equipment, it is imperative that you locate a supplier who is interested in supplying the right equipment that you need without extras that you do not need. A helpful, concerned medical supply salesperson will ask you many questions which will help in selecting the right equipment. If you are not asked questions about your family member's ability or disability, size, weight, age, or prognosis, you can be assured that they are either not that interested in supplying the correct equipment, or do not have the experience to help guide you in your selections. In either case, go to another supplier. Let me give you an example. Did you know that wheelchairs come in many sizes and models? Standard adult wheelchairs have an 18" wide seat. The same model with removable arms will give the person almost 2" additional seating area. A narrow adult chair with removable arms has just about the same seat area as a standard 18" chair. Some wheelchairs have fixed footrests, while others have removable or swing away foot rests. A removable armrest and removable footrest is absolutely necessary to achieve a safe transfer of the person from chair to bed or from chair to commode, wheelchair to car. Some wheelchairs will go through bathroom or bedroom doorways and some will not. Obviously you need an expert so you get the correct and most efficient equipment.

It is important to select a supplier that has a considerable variety of equipment for you to see at the time of purchase. To again use our wheelchair example, if the supplier has only one or two sizes or models to choose from it may not be possible to get the one best model or size for your family member. There will be times when one piece of equipment will not be adequate for all occurrences. For example, a wheelchair that will go through the bathroom door may be too small for the person's comfort and support during other times the chair will be used, and so the chair's ability to go through the bathroom door will become secondary to the other times the person will be using the chair. Perhaps it will be necessary to obtain a smaller transfer chair or a shower-commode chair for use when transportation to the bathroom is necessary.

Inquire about the repair facilities at the medical supply store. In time, your equipment will need repair work, and it is important that the supplier selling the equipment is able to repair it in a timely fashion. Will the supplier loan you equipment while yours is being repaired? Does the supplier maintain an adequate supply of parts? Asking these questions at the time of purchase or rental can prevent problems for you and your family member in the future.

If you are purchasing equipment in anticipation of the return of your family member from the hospital or rehabilitation center, ask if the equipment be returned for a full refund if it is found that the person just cannot use the equipment, or doesn't like it. Of course, you must be reasonable about such a request, as you cannot expect a supplier to accept a return after the equipment has been used for several days by the person. I am sure you realize that some medical supply items cannot be returned due to health regulations that cover items placed next to the body.

Let me give you a few thoughts and ideas about some of the more common items you may need to obtain. Walkers are often necessary for your family member to safely ambulate. A standard walker will do fine in the home, but if the person using it will be able to go out in the car, either now or as their health improves, a folding walker should be considered as it is impossible to get a standard walker in even the largest car trunk. If your family member has suffered a stroke, or if one arm is considerably stronger than the other, a hemi-walker or pyramid cane may be considered.

Quad canes (a cane with four feet) are available with either a large or small base. In most cases, the larger base will give considerably more stability and is usually the preferred size. The supplier or therapist will assist you in setting the quad cane to the proper height, as this is most important to obtain maximize utilization of the cane.

Bath benches or shower benches should be adjustable in height for maximum utilization and safety. If the person is somewhat unstable, consider the bench with a back for greater security and comfort, or one with a back that conventionally clamps on the side of the tub. The bathroom can be a dangerous place for anyone with decreased strength and/or endurance. It is important to make the bathroom as safe as possible by installing properly placed wall-mounted grab bars, tub-mounted grab bars and bath transfer benches clamped to the edge of the tub, elevated toilet seats, and toilet assist rails. Your medical supply store should demonstrate this equipment, make recommendations, and explain its use.

To facilitate the care of your family member and to avoid injury to yourself, a hospital bed may be needed. Hospital beds come with a variety of functions. Some are electrically controlled — some are manual (crank). Both come with the following features:

• Head up, foot up. This is a manual or semi-electric bed.

• Head up, foot up, bed up. (The entire bed can be raised up from the floor). This is a full electric or three crank manual bed.

If your family member is independent in getting in and out of bed and requires no bed care, a manual bed or an electric bed with head up, foot up bed will be more than adequate.

If the family member needs moderate to maximal assistance in getting out of and into bed, and requires any bed care, a full electric bed will be essential.

If your family member will be confined to a bed or a wheelchair or perhaps both, it is important to have the proper body support that can be obtained by a water or alternating pressure air mattress for the bed, and a flotation cushion for the wheelchair. Using the proper support can greatly add to comfort as well as prevent bed sores. Your durable medical supplier can help you in making the proper selections.

As new advances are made in medicine each year, the number of senior citizens in our country increases. New developments in equipment will be seen in many of the larger durable medical supply stores, making life more comfortable and rewarding for our seniors, and others as well. Power lift and recline chairs have made life much more comfortable for people with arthritis and others who find it difficult to reach a standing position from a comfortable chair. Under certain conditions, Medicare and other insurers will help pay for a portion of such equipment if the medical need is documented by your physician. Three wheeled electric scooters have given mobility to many persons previously confined to a small area in a wheelchair. I strongly advise you to shop carefully for this type of equipment, and buy only from those suppliers that have the equipment to try in the store. Be sure the supplier is able to maintain the equipment with trained repair persons, and understand the guarantee that comes with each product. To buy such equipment, which in time will surely need some service work, from mail order organizations or from TV advertisements will surely end with major problems when service or repair is needed.

Some family members will need orthopedic support products in addition to the durable medical supplies. Not all medical suppliers are able to offer this service, however, they will be able to direct you to a supplier than can offer this service. Orthopedic supports should be supplied and fitted by a trained, certified fitter. Do not hesitate to ask if their fitters are certified to properly fit surgical appliances. Proper fitting is an absolute necessity if the appliance is to do the job it is intended to do. A good orthopedic supply store will be willing to make a house call to do the fitting if your family member is unable to come to the supply store. There will, of course, be an added cost for such a service.

For most of us purchasing medical equipment, the cost of the equipment can be an important consideration. It is just as foolish to buy the cheapest you can find as it is to buy the very best that is available to you. The older, mainly house-bound wheelchair person will do nicely with a moderately priced wheelchair. The younger, more active person will need a stronger, more durable wheelchair. A reliable durable medical supplier truly interested in you and your family member will help you with your selection, and if cost is one of your major concerns be sure your supplier knows this.

To buy the equipment or to rent the equipment — a decision that must be made. There are many factors that must be considered when making this decision, especially if most or some of the cost will be covered by Medicare or other insurance carrier. Although Medicare regulations are subject to frequent change, these regulations usually require the rental of the more expensive durable medical equipment such as hospital beds and wheelchairs. At present, Medicare will pay 80% of the approved rental amount, and the person, or the person and a secondary insurer, will be responsible for the balance of the rental cost. Less expensive equipment such as commodes or walkers can be either purchased or rented. Let your equipment supplier help you with this decision, but as a general rule, if the equipment will be used for a short recovery time, rental may be best for you. If the expected need for the equipment will be for a considerable length of time, purchase may be best.

There could well be a situation that you are unable to decide which would be the wiser decision, to buy or to rent. Ask your supplier if it is possible to rent the equipment for a short period of time before making the final decision, and then applying the rental cost to the purchase of the equipment. Many medical suppliers will be willing to exchange the rental equipment for new equipment should you decide to purchase. In some instances, you may be able to purchase the rental equipment at a reduced rate at the end of the first month's rental. You should discuss this at the time of the rental.

When you are caring for someone at home, you will have little time to call your own. The paperwork relating to rental or purchase of equipment can many times be very difficult, confusing, and time consuming. To the durable medical supplier, this paperwork is routine and the supplier understands the system and its many complexities. In selecting a supplier, select one that will submit the necessary paperwork to Medicare for you, and send you a copy of all submissions he has made. Some insurance companies will only pay the person for medical equipment, and these requests for payment must be submitted by the person or someone responsible for this paperwork. Your supplier should be willing to assist you in completing insurance claims if you are unable to do so. Questions relating to Medicare or other third party payers should be asked when discussing the equipment with your supplier.

If you have been trading with a specific durable medical equipment supplier and feel that you are not getting the services that you need, even if you have this equipment in your home on a rental basis, shop around and find a new supplier. Don't hesitate to call your present supplier, tell them you are switching firms and ask them to remove the equipment. Never feel trapped into keeping a supplier and paying them your money, if you are dissatisfied.

In summary, consider these aspects in selecting a durable medical supplier:

• Does the supplier maintain a well-rounded stock from which to choose your equipment?

• Does the supplier maintain a repair department?

• Is the supplier, manager, or sales person knowledgeable about the equipment and its uses?

• Does the salesperson ask questions about your family member to better understand your needs?

• Does the supplier have a reasonable return policy?

• Does the supplier have a trained orthopedic fitter if needed?

• Is the supplier willing to explain the various insurance plans?

• Is the supplier willing to assist you in processing Medicare or other insurance claims?

• Is the supplier willing to rent as well as sell or combine rental with the option to buy?

• Is the supplier willing to give you the time and attention you need if you are only making inquiries about his supplies?

Caring for a Person in Bed

The personal care of an individual at home should be tailored to meet the specific needs of each person. It may help at times to ask yourself how you would feel in that person's place, because the difficult times often come up when the person has lost independence and must stay in bed. Coping with the losses and still maintaining one's self-esteem can be a challenge. Accepting what the person can do to help themselves will also help you to be more sensitive to their feelings.

One way to allow the person to express a degree of control is to include them in as much of their personal care as possible, even if all they can do is wash their face. Also, always tell the person what you are doing and give them every opportunity to make decisions and choices. This gives the person a sense of control. (Above all, when the situation presents itself, challenge the person.) You may find that at times the person can do more than anyone thought possible.

At best, the information you may get from the hospital or doctor on how to care for a bedbound person may be scanty. There are many things to remember and learn about caring for a bedbound person. This chapter will provide you with straightforward advice and a step-by-step process to follow, including the equipment and supplies you will need. Some precautions and special considerations will also be included. Let us start with bed positioning.

Positioning

Proper positioning is the first and most important aspect of caring for the person that you will need to learn. All other activity will depend on good positioning. Proper positioning will facilitate caring for the person and encourage their increased level of independence and achievement. Combining ease for the caregiver, comfort for the person, and safety for all will be a real learning process for both of you.

List of Supplies/Equipment

• Drawsheet or fabric incontinence (waterproof) pad

• Footboard

• Flexible back support (if regular bed is used)

• 3-4 pillows

• Neck pillow (optional)

• Bedside table

When lying in bed for long periods of time, proper positioning is necessary to prevent bedsores (decubiti), loss of flexibility of joints, and tightness (contractures) of the muscles. These conditions can happen in a short time and cause unremitting pain for the person and increased personal care for you as the caregiver. Once you have practiced techniques to prevent these problems, they will become part of your routine.

There are several different types of special mattresses which may help to prevent the problems of bedsores and pain. Water mattresses are available for under $100 in medical supply stores, and people from these stores will install them on request. Egg-crate or foam mattresses are often given to patients when they are in the hospital, and you can bring these mattresses home when the person is discharged. No matter what kind of mattress you have, it will be necessary to change the person's position every two hours or so. You will find what is best for the person and what repositioning schedule can fit into your daily routine.

The person's bed should be accessible from both sides. Whether the bed is a full electric type or manual, the height should be raised to the highest level. This will help to reduce strain on your back as you care for the person in bed.

If you have a hospital bed, the person's position should be high enough toward the head of the bed to allow the head or foot of the bed to be elevated properly. In other words, when you raise the foot of the bed, the bed should bend at the person's knees. When you raise the head of the bed, the bed should bend near the person's hips. If you do not have a hospital bed, the person should be positioned so that you can properly raise the legs or head with pillows and still have equal room on all sides of the person. This proper bed positioning is important because adequate postural support is crucial in order to stay in one position for any length of time, or in order to be positioned for participation in activities.

Moving the Person Up in Bed

1. Make sure the height of the bed is appropriate for your height so as to eliminate your having to bend over excessively.

2. Lower the head of the bed until it is flat.

3. The person can assist by bending knees and placing feet flat on the bed. If he/she cannot keep feet in this position, prop them up in place with a pillow.

4. Place one arm under the person's shoulders and one under their knees.

5. Straighten your back and bend your knees, standing with feet more than a shoulder's width apart. You will be using your thigh muscles and shifting your weight from one leg to the other on the movement.

6. Instruct the person to press their heels into the mattress as you lift toward the head of the bed.

7. Count to three, out loud, so you and the person know when to move together.

It may take more than one time and this is fine. Repeat the process until the person reaches the desired height in bed. If a drawsheet is available you may hold the corners on one side and maintain the proper position of your back and feet. Follow the same directions and change from one side to the other of the bed until the person is in the proper location.

Now that the person is at the proper place high in the bed, you can continue with other positioning techniques.

Alignment of Person in Bed

1. Observe person from the foot of the bed. The shoulders, hips, and feet should be in a straight line while the person is lying in a supine position (on their back).

2. If the shoulders are not aligned with the hips, put your one hand under the shoulder blade and the other on top of the shoulder you want to reposition. Gently pull it into position.

3. The hips can be realigned in the same manner with one hand under the lower back/buttocks and the other on top of the hip you are moving. Gently pull the hips toward you.

4. Both feet should be positioned with special attention to the back of the heels, which is an area where breakdown of the skin easily occurs. Place a small roll (a good sized hand towel) under the spot where the leg and foot meet (Achilles tendon area) to raise the heels off of the bed. If the person moves their legs around in bed you may want to consider trying fleece-lined booties on their feet. The feet should be propped up in dorsiflexion (bent up, toes pointing to the ceiling) with a pillow rolled behind them to maintain the position. This is necessary to prevent foot drop. When one spends a great deal of time in bed, the feet may tend to drop to the point where they are

almost in line with the legs. This causes the Achilles tendon to shorten and makes normal walking and even simple transfers difficult, if not impossible. A footboard will prevent the linens from bending the toes downward and the person from going too low in the bed.

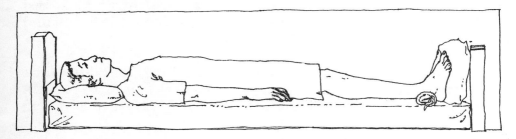

5. Now go to the end of the bed again. Are the shoulders, hips, and feet aligned properly? Now ask the person if he or she is comfortable.

Elevating the Head of the Bed

1. Is the person high enough in the bed?

2. When elevating the head of the bed do so slowly, in gradual increments, especially if the person has not been sitting up for long periods of time. A back support with pillow can be used for a regular bed.

3. Arrange pillows behind neck or try pulling them down under the shoulders. This is the best time to try the neck pillow or a large towel roll to align the person's head.

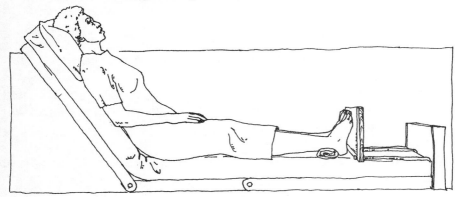

Elevating Foot of Bed

1. Check to see if person is high enough in bed.

2. Elevate the foot of the bed gradually until both knees are flexed (bent) and fully supported by the mattress. In a regular bed you can do this by placing 1-2 pillows under the knees and placing both feet flat on the bed.

    This position is important in maintaining flexibility of the person's hips and knees. Pillows can also be used to prevent both legs from rotating outward or inward toward each other.

The Sidelying Position

    This can be a most desirable way for the person to rest and often is the position of choice for sleep. It is excellent for prevention of bedsores developing along the spine or buttocks.

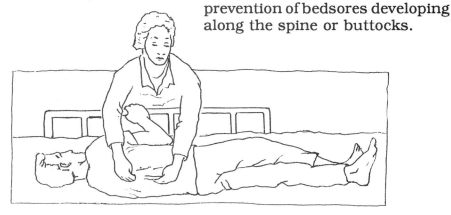

1. Observe person in bed for proper placement. He or she should be in the middle of the bed.

2. Check to see that the height of the bed is appropriate.

3. Put up the siderail on the side the person is turning to. This will assist with movement if the person can grab hold of it, and will also provide for safety.

4. Locate yourself beside the person in the middle of the length of the bed.

5. Place one hand on the person's shoulder blade nearest to you and the other hand on the small of the back close to the buttocks.

6. Gently roll the person towards you, keeping the knee flexed so it crosses over the other leg. A drawsheet can be used to facilitate turning the person also. Just pick up the corners of this pad and roll the person over, allowing the knee to flex.

7. Prop a double rolled pillow behind the back from the shoulders to the hips to help maintain the person's position.

8. Next, check the person's alignment as you stand at the foot of the bed. The shoulders, hips, and feet should be in a straight line.

9. If the shoulder next to the bed needs adjusting, go to the side of the bed where the person is facing. Put one hand on top of that shoulder, put the other under the shoulder blade, and gently pull it toward you.

10. The procedure for straightening the hips can be done from behind the person. Place one hand under the hip and the other hand on top of the other hip. Gently pull person's hips toward you.

11. Bring both feet up in a flexed (bent) position. A pillow or towel roll can be used to keep the feet this way.

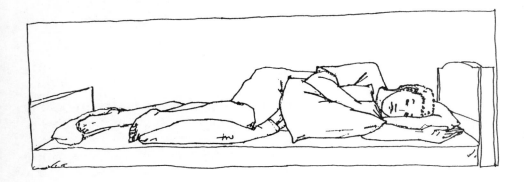

12. Check areas where skin is in contact with other bony areas such as ankles and knees. Also, check the position of the hip on top as it is usually on a decline; this adds extra pressure on the pelvis, which can be most uncomfortable.

13. Place a pillow between the knees and ankles which will also lift the top hip into proper alignment. The person's knees should be bent comfortably and flexion of both feet can be maintained by a towel roll or pillow propped in place. This step will reduce friction on bony areas and aid in the prevention of bedsores.

Securing Bedpan Under Person

The bedpan needs to be positioned properly in order to keep bed linens clean and reduce the caregiver's workload. Also, it can be embarrassing for the person to have someone very close by while the person evacuates their bowels, so be sensitive to the need for privacy.

Supplies/Equipment

- Bedpan
- Toilet paper
- 2 chux, or blue pads
- Clean, wet washcloth
- Towel
- Drape to cover person

- Uniwash/Unicare, Periwash/Pericare, or similar product

Procedure

1. Wash your hands.

2. Lower head and foot of bed. Check person's position in bed. Is he/she up high enough to raise head of bed comfortably?

3. Pull the side rail up on the side of the bed that you are turning the person toward.

4. Place yourself on the opposite side of the bed.

5. Put one hand under the shoulder blade and one under the knee nearest you.

6. Gently roll the person over, flexing the top knee over the bottom one to maintain this position.

7. Place chux or blue pad under the person's buttocks across the width of the bed to protect the linens, if one is not in place already.

8. Position the bedpan next to the buttocks assuring enough of the pan is located between his or her legs.

9. With one hand under the knees and the other securing the pan in place, turn person back toward you and onto the bedpan. Use a drape over the person to maintain dignity.

10. Raise the head of the bed as high as possible, to simulate a sitting position.

11. Flex the knees and place both feet flat on bed, if desired.

12. Make sure the person is comfortable and excuse yourself for a short time to give the person more privacy. Pull up the other side rail on bed if you leave. (Before removing the bedpan, you may pour water over the pubic area for cleansing purposes.)

13. To remove the bedpan, lower head of bed, place one hand on the knees, roll the person over, and secure the bedpan with the other hand.

14. Roll person off of the bedpan. Remove the bedpan and put a chux over it until you clean up the person.

15. Wash and dry the area around the perineum and the rectum well. A skin cleanser or lotion such as Periwash/Pericare or Uniwash/Unicare can be used to prevent skin breakdown which can be caused by urine or feces. This is an excellent time to give the person a relaxing backrub.

16. Return person to a comfortable position and clean up bedpan.

17. Wash your hands and allow the person to wash up also.

The Bed Bath

This can be time well spent with the person, time in which to enjoy each other's company. It is good to set aside enough time so as not to rush and to allow him or her to be involved as much as possible. Throughout the following steps the maintenance of the person's dignity should be a major issue.

Ask anyone else in the room to leave.

Supplies/Equipment

• Bath Basin (1 or 2)*

• Light blanket or sheet

• Soap or bath oil

• 1-2 towels

• Washcloth

• Deodorant

• Skin lotion

• Chux, or blue pad

• Toothbrush

• Toothpaste

• Mouthwash

• Small basin (or bowl)

• Bedside table or dresser for equipment

* You may use one basin and change water frequently, or use one for washing and one for rinsing.

Range of motion exercises can be incorporated into bath time. Read about how to guide the joints through active, passive, or active assistive range of motion later in this chapter.

Procedure

1. Wash your hands.

2. Tell the person your plan.

3. Adjust the height of the bed so it is appropriate for you.

4. Allow the person to do what he or she can independently and to be part of all decisions.

5. Offer a urinal or bedpan before starting the bath (directions on previous pages).

6. Although oral care can be done upon awakening in morning or before breakfast, offer it again at this time. If the person has dentures, you may choose to wash them in the sink.

7. Start with towel under chin and with head of bed elevated. Give the person a sip of water before brushing the teeth.

8. Offer a small basin or bowl for the person to spit into during brushing and sips of water to rinse the mouth. Empty the basin or bowl while you fill the large basin with bath water.

9. Make sure the bath water temperature is comfortable for the person.

10. Remove his/her bed clothes and drape a light blanket or sheet for privacy.

11. Place a towel under chin/neck.

12. Wash the eyes without soap on the washcloth, starting with the inner eye working toward the outer eye. Change each section of the washcloth used for each eye.

13. If the person uses soap on his or her face, use it sparingly on washcloth and finish the face, neck, and ears.

14. Rinse thoroughly and dry by patting gently.

15. Remove only the parts of the drape that expose the body part you will be washing immediately.

16. Start with the drape across chest and the towel under the arm, farthest from you first.

17. Wash each arm from wrist to shoulder, including the underarm area. Place each hand in the basin to soak, if possible. Use smooth, even strokes and support the elbows at all times. Check any bony areas for redness or broken skin.

18. Rinse, dry, and apply deodorant and/or powder. Repeat the process on the other arm.

19. Remove the drape to expose the chest. Wash, dry, and rinse thoroughly.

20. Keep the towel over the chest area and lower the drape to expose the abdomen.

21. Wash, rinse, and dry the abdomen, then re-cover the person with the drape.

22. Uncover the person's leg farthest from you and put a towel under it. Bend the knee, supporting it, and have the person maintain this position if possible.

23. Wash from ankle to hip gently and evenly. Rinse, dry, and cover the leg while soaking foot in basin. Repeat this for the leg nearest you.

24. Do not massage the legs unless you have checked with the physician first. Bony prominences such as knees and ankle bones should be checked and lotion applied, especially if area is dry or irritated. Areas of broken skin should be brought to a doctor's attention.

25. Change the bath water and check the temperature for person's comfort.

26. Position the person on the side away from you. Place a towel on the bed slightly under the back. Wash and dry the back and buttocks from the shoulders down. This is the time for a back rub to promote relaxation and to prevent skin breakdown. Put lotion on your hands and rub over the skin using a circular motion. Start at sacral area (lower back) and work upwards on either side of the spine in a fan-out motion. Be aware of any red or irritated areas; massage in that specific place to reduce the chance of skin breakdown.

27. Wash and dry the rectal area from front to back. Rinse and dry well.

28. Return the person to a back-lying position and put the drape in place.

29. Change the bath water.

30. Bathe the genital area, exposing only the part to be washed by placing a towel over the chest. Wash from front to back using a different section of the washcloth for each stroke. Give special attention to folds of skin; i.e., if the person is not circumcised, gently pull the foreskin covering the head of the penis back to expose the entire head of the penis. Gently wash this area.

31. If an indwelling catheter is in place, wash the place of contact with skin well, rinse, and dry. Place a perineal pad or scrotal support at this time.

32. Put on clean bed clothes, eye glasses, watch, or other articles worn by person daily.

33. Place a towel underneath the person's head and brush/comb hair.

34. Change the bed linen and apply chux or blue pad as needed under the person. To change linen when the person is in bed, roll him or her to one side of the bed. Tuck dirty linen under the person and put clean sheets in place halfway, folding them under the soiled linen. Then turn the person to the other side

over the mound of dirty and clean sheets. Pull the sheets through and finish making the bed. If the sheets are soiled when you start, use a chux or blue pad between the dirty and clean linen to keep the clean linen from getting soiled in the process of making the bed.

35. Put the siderails in place and make sure the person is comfortable.

The use of powder is optional, but it is best to remember not to use powder until the skin is dry. Do not use large amounts or combine powder with use of lotions or oils. The combinations of items can irritate the skin. If the person wears elastic or surgical stockings, never use oils or powders because it reduces the elasticity of the stockings.

Bath oil can be used often or occasionally for dry or irritated skin sometimes caused by use of too much soap. You do not have to rinse when using bath oil.

Initially this process may take considerable time, but as you become more familiar with the bathing techniques, you will develop your own style, allowing a more efficient use of time and a plan that best suits you and the person for whom you are caring.

Dressing Changes

If this is new to you, be sure to observe the dressing change in the hospital before your loved one goes home. This gives you an opportunity to ask any questions or voice any concerns you may have about the wound. Make sure that you have a place available near the bed for your supplies and that area is well lit, ventilated, and private. The person should be in a comfortable position and the time should be appropriate (not near meal time). Usually after the bath is a convenient time. Should the person require a sterile dressing technique, contact a doctor or visiting nurse.

Supplies/Equipment

• Latex examination gloves

• Sterile dressing tray. This tray will come with sterile gloves, forceps, 4 x 4 dressings and it can be purchased at your local durable medical supply company and some drugstores.

• Cleaning solution — if ordered by physician

• Skin prep pads

• Tape

• Plastic bag for soiled dressings

Procedure

1. Explain your plan to the person.

2. Position and drape the person.

3. Adjust the bed to a height appropriate for you.

4. Wash your hands and put on examination gloves.

5. Remove the old dressings and place in garbage bag. Tie the ends and place in garbage pail.

6. Remove gloves and wash your hands.

7. Open the sterile dressing tray and spread the outside wrap. Take special care to touch only tips and outer exterior surfaces.

8. Open all dressings and drop them onto the sterile field.

9. Put on the sterile gloves.

10. Clean wound as directed by physician/nurse.

11. Use the forceps (tweezers) to handle dressings and while placing them over wound.

12. Apply skin prep to any skin which will be in contact with the tape. Let it dry.

13. Tape the dressing in place.

14. Wash your hands after removing your supplies and gloves.

Bedsores

Bedsores are the layman's term for pressure sores or decubitus ulcers. It is an area of skin that has been injured or traumatized. Initially, a bedsore will appear as a red area which does not fade or disappear after the pressure to the spot has been relieved. Usually within twenty minutes after a position change, the redness should disappear. Gentle massage with lotion in a circular motion around the reddened area can help increase blood supply to the spot. If after twenty minutes the area is still red, a bedsore may be developing. The skin may break or blister next or a small open sore may be seen. A decubitus ulcer can become an open wound that may drain and reach deep tissues or bone.

A sore can develop if the skin is subject to pressure over an extended period of time. Any restriction of movement that decreases blood supply can produce this situation. The best way to decrease the chance of developing a bedsore is to keep moving. This can be done by the person or the caregiver. Later in this chapter you will learn range of motion exercises which will increase movement for a bedbound person. The important part to remember is that any bedbound person is at high risk for a bedsore. Poor nutrition, skin condition (too dry or too moist), and certain diseases also increase a person's risk factors, in addition to immobility.

Circulatory problems, phlebitis, diabetes, anemia, or any condition that reduces a person's sensation of pain or pressure, as well as an inability to move can increase the chance that a bedsore will develop. A confused or unconscious person is a likely candidate to develop bedsores since they may not be able to indicate or react to a problem. Also, a frequently wet or soiled person can easily develop these sores.

The bony prominences are the areas most susceptible to breakdown. The skin over the bony areas are: the back of the head, shoulder blades, spine, elbows, buttocks, hips, thighs, knees, ankles, and heels. Again, positioning is most important, as is checking closely any point where skin is in contact with a catheter. Sores can develop behind the ears when oxygen tubing is worn. A cast or splint can also cause sores.

The prevention of bedsores must be a part of the care you provide and you will automatically learn to check all the specified areas and skin in general as you become more familiar with caregiving techniques. You will definitely want to spare the person the pain of a bedsore and yourself another worry.

The best prevention is movement, and frequent positioning may be the most effective way to assure good skin integrity. Change position every two hours during waking hours. During the night, you can change the person's position less frequently, but always reposition if the person awakens during the night. Proper positioning and movement in bed is of utmost importance because if done improperly these activities may increase the chance of skin breakdown. A shearing movement can occur whenever a person is moved in bed. This happens when the skin over bony prominences does not move as the person is being moved or positioned. This shearing movement must be avoided at all times, as this causes a large percentage of bedsores. Whenever you roll, turn, or lift a person, never slide or drag them across a surface too fast or without telling them when you are going to proceed. Increased friction occurs as the skin comes into contact with linens and can cause this shearing movement. Always gently lift using care to move slowly and using proper technique to prevent problems for yourself and the person.

Specific equipment can be beneficial in prevention of bedsores also. A water or air mattress are often used for people who spend much of their time in bed to reduce the effects of immobility. A trapeze bar can be a useful piece of equipment in prevention of shearing movements because the person can assist in lifting and positioning in bed.

One of the best ways to impress upon yourself to check the pressure spots is to be consciously aware of how you lie in bed and what bony prominences would be most prone to breakdown on yourself.

The care of a bedsore can be as varied as these sores themselves. It is best to check with your doctor, occupational or physical therapist, or home care nurse for direction. Meanwhile, you can keep linens dry and free of wrinkles, massage skin over bony areas for three to five minutes every two hours when positioning. Do range of motion along with increasing frequency of positioning. Also, encourage adequate fluid intake and proper nutrition as measures to prevent bedsores.

Feeding and Eating in Bed

This can be one of the most enjoyable times you spend with the person all day. People often share how their day has gone or tell a joke during mealtimes. Conversation should center around pleasant topics. Because people with a decreased activity level often have less of an appetite, food should be presented in small servings so as not to overwhelm them. The dining atmosphere should be as pleasant as possible, using appropriate lighting and, perhaps, some soft music. All of these ideas may positively influence a person's appetite, however, considerations to past dietary preferences and routines should also be part of your plan for mealtime. The person's level of independence should also be taken into consideration, and plenty of time should be allowed for the person to eat at his or her own pace. Of course, if the person can eat independently, they should be encouraged to do so.

Supplies/Equipment

• Chair for yourself

• Bedside table or lap tray

• Utensils

• Napkin

• Towel

• Straw or travel cup with lid to prevent spills

Procedure

1. Wash your hands.

2. Position the person in bed comfortably with their head elevated. Ideally, the person should be in a position as close to sitting as possible. The head should be well supported, not tilted to either side, backward, or forward, to prevent swallowing or choking problems.

3. Place the food between yourselves so he or she can see it. Let the person decide in what order they would like to eat the food.

4. Put a napkin under his or her chin or spread towel on lap.

5. Begin to feed the person with a fork or spoon. Only fill halfway to prevent spills.

6. Offer fluids every few bites, or as the person indicates.

7. Remove the food and tray when finished.

8. Wash the person's hands and mouth if they are unable to do so.

9. Keep record of fluid intake if directed by physician. If person is not hungry when you present the meal, remove it and try later. Smaller amounts may also help.

Range of Motion Exercises

The degree of movement in which a joint rotates or revolves is the range of motion (ROM) of that joint. Persons who have a limitation of any movement or who must spend time being inactive can become weak and lose strength and/or endurance in a short time. In order to prevent the problems associated with disuse of muscles and contracture formation, a person and/or caregiver will be told to do range of motion exercises. It is best to check with the person's physician and therapist for any contraindications. An occupational or physical therapist can design a plan for the individual person upon recommendation from the physician.

Including range of motion exercises in the person's daily plan will help to increase or maintain function of a joint and muscles as well as increasing or maintaining muscle tone and strength. These exercises will encourage independence and can be achieved by involving the person in activities of daily living such as washing his/her face, eating, using a trapeze, or getting in and out of bed. The level to which a person may need assistance with performing these movements can vary. Some persons will need passive range of motion in which a caregiver performs the movements for the person. Active assistive range of motion means the person and caregiver together move the joint through the range of motion. If the person can do the exercises independently, this is called active range of motion. A person can start out needing passive range of motion and move onto active assistive and eventually be able to do active range of motion independently. If you know the person's level of need and tolerance to exercise, this is a good place to start.

Some important things to remember are:

• These exercises should not be done without the person's knowledge or compliance if possible.

• Remember to set the bed to appropriate height for yourself and make sure the person is comfortable.

• Always support a joint and never allow quick or jerky movements.

• Never force or push a joint beyond its limits or cause pain.

• Use smooth, slow, and gentle movements and continue until resistance is met.

• When performing range of motion, watch the person's face closely for any indication of pain. A grimace or vocal warning may be the response to tell you to stop.

• Start with three completions of range of motion for each joint. Build up to twenty times each, if tolerated by the person.

Shoulder Exercise 1

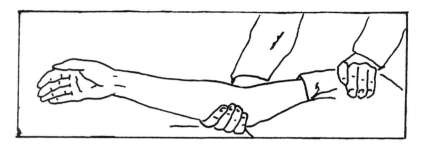

Put arm at side. Hold the elbow with one hand and place the other hand on the shoulder.

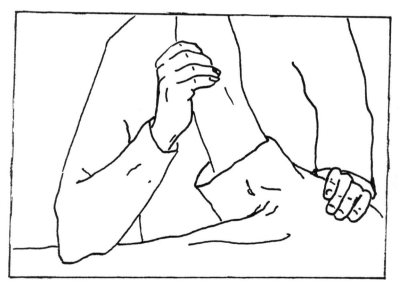

Bring arm straight up and then return it to the bed.

Shoulder Exercise 2

Person lying on back. Put arm on bed away from body with elbow bent. Put your hand on the person's upper arm near the elbow and grasp person's hand.

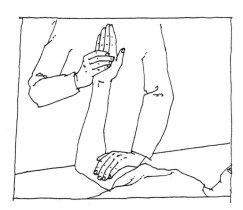

Move forearm down, palm towards the bed.

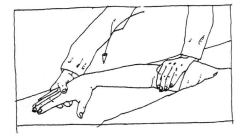

Return forearm to original position, then move back in the other direction.

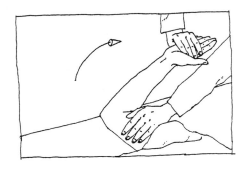

Shoulder Exercise 3

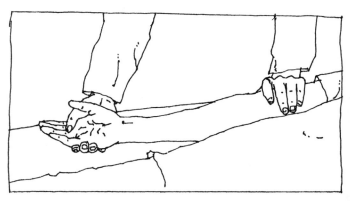

Put arm at side. Keep arm straight. Put one hand just above the elbow and the other hand in their hand.

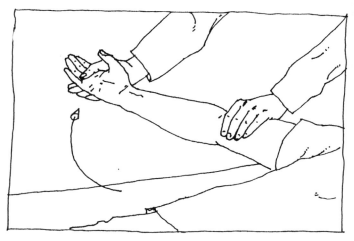

Move the entire arm away from the body and then return it to the side of their body.

Elbow Exercise

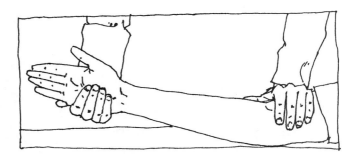

Put arm at side. Grasp the hand in one hand and support the upper arm just above the elbow.

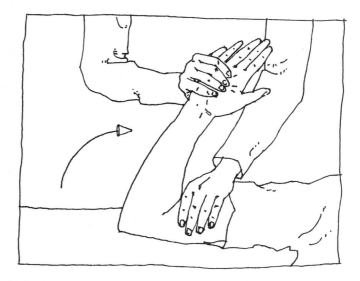

Hold the forearm on the bed. Bring the hand towards the shoulder, then return the arm to the bed.

Forearm Exercise

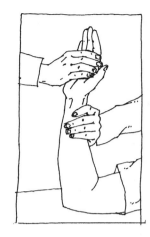

Put upper arm next to the body. Bend the elbow so that the hand is pointed to the ceiling.

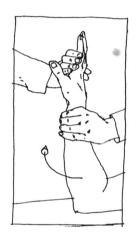

Turn the hand away from the face.

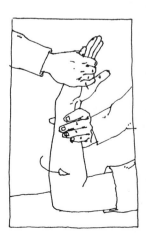

Turn the hand towards the face.

Wrist Exercise 1

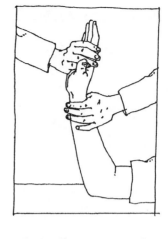

Place the person's upper arm next to their body. Bend the elbow so that the hand is pointing to the ceiling. Grasp the person's forearm just above the wrist with one hand. Then grasp their palm, holding the fingers straight and together.

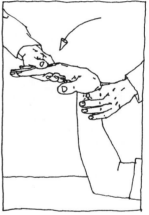

Bend the wrist down, palm down.

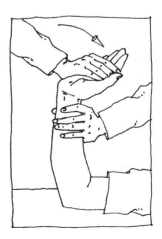

Bend the wrist in the other direction, palm up.

Wrist Exercise 2

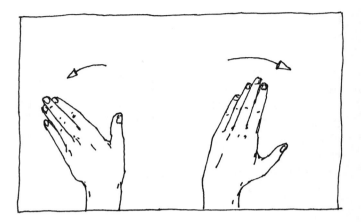

Hold the forearm straight. Move the hand from side to side.

Finger Exercise 1

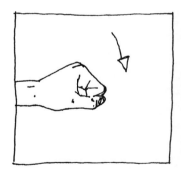

Clench the person's fist.

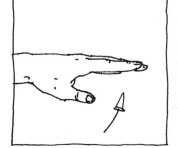

Bring the fingers out straight.

Finger Exercise 2

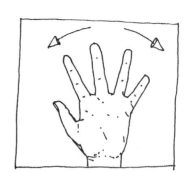

Move the fingers apart from one another.

Bring the fingers back together.

Finger Exercise 3

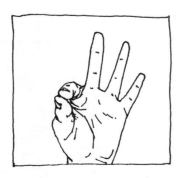 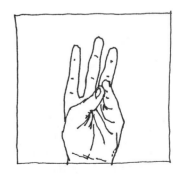

Bring thumb and tip of each finger together.

Hip and Knee Exercise 1

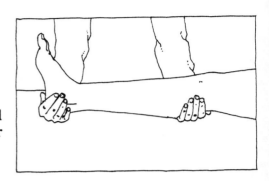

Support the leg – one hand cupping the ankle and the other hand just below the knee.

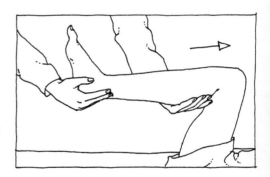

Move the leg towards the hip.

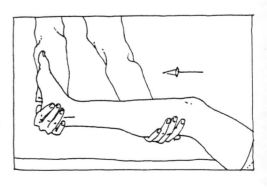

Return the leg to bed, so that the leg is straight again (as in the first picture).

Hip and Knee Exercise 2

Support the leg, holding it straight – one hand under the knee and the other hand under the heel.

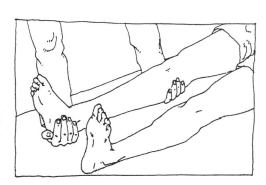

Move the entire leg away from the body.

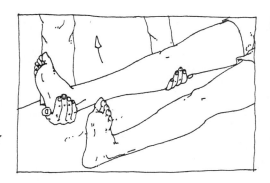

Return the straight leg to the center of the body.

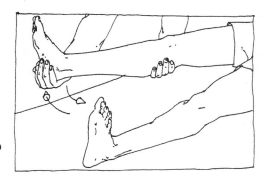

Hip and Knee Exercise 3

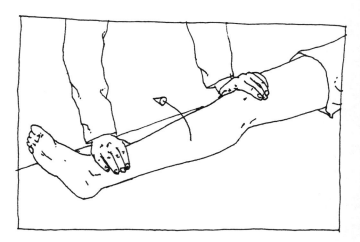

Grasp the knee and the ankle on the top. Roll the entire leg outwards.

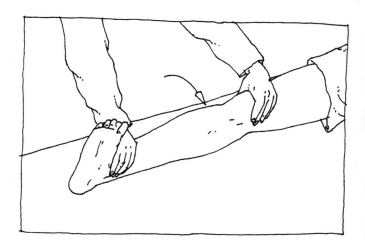

Roll the entire leg inwards.

Ankle Exercise

Place the leg straight out on the bed. Put one hand just above the ankle and the other hand on the sole of the foot by the instep.

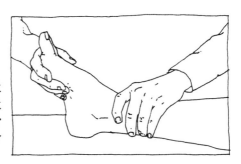

Gently push the foot upwards towards the person's face.

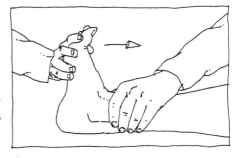

Gently push the foot back towards the foot of the bed.

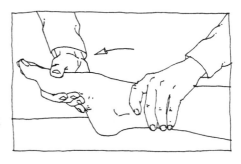

Foot Exercise

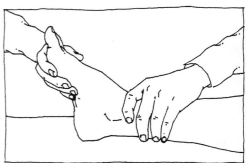

Place one hand on the sole of the foot by the instep.

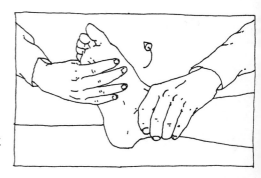

Move the sole of the foot inwards.

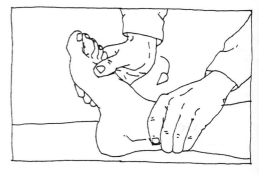

Move the sole of the foot outwards, away from the body.

Toe Exercise

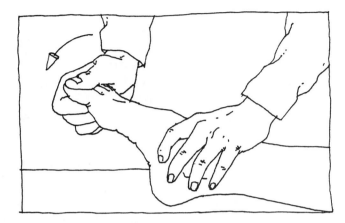

Gently move toes toward the sole of the foot.

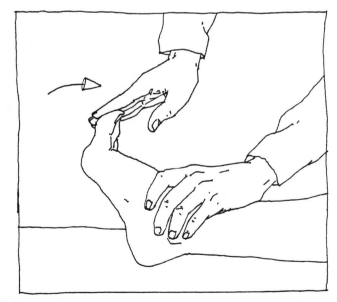

Gently straighten toes back to the normal position and then towards the knee.

Head Exercise 1

Put the head of the bed up or prop the person up in bed with pillows. Support the chin and back of the head. Move the head back and then forwards, chin to chest.

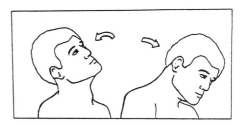

Head Exercise 2

Support the chin and back of the head. Move the head to the right and then to the left, chin to shoulder on each side.

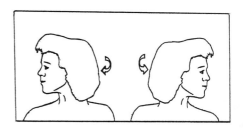

Head Exercise 3

Support the head on each temple. Gently move the head to the right, then to the left, ear to shoulder on each side.

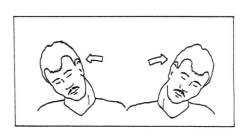

The head, neck, and shoulder blade muscles become tight very quickly when a person is unable to move independently. These limitations of movement will hamper many activities, even bathing, so it is especially important to exercise these areas, along with other joints, as indicated. The most important thing to remember is not to force a joint to move. Gentle, smooth motion is the best way to perform the movements and protect the joints.

Now proceed to the other side of the bed and starting at the shoulder repeat the same movements. It may seem to take a great deal of time to learn all of these exercises, but if you practice on yourself in bed before you go to sleep at night it will become familiar much sooner.

As you become more proficient in your caregiving role, and you will, not only will the time you spend decrease, but also the stress or anxiety you feel will also diminish. A sense of humor can be a most important part of coping with the stress and allows you and the person to reduce the anxiety together and even have fun!

Although this chapter discusses how the caregiver is to do range of motion exercises for the person in bed, whenever possible, have the person do the exercises out of bed, either independently or with as little assistance as possible.

7

Transfers

Transfers, the moving of a person from one place to another, are frequently considered by caregivers to be the area of greatest concern in caring for another person. Some common concerns of caregivers include:

• Fear of hurting the person.

• Fear of hurting themselves, especially their back.

• Fear of not being able to get the person back to bed, after they have been transferred out of bed.

• Fear of letting the person fall to the floor.

These fears are often shared by the person being transferred, as well. As a result, many weak, elderly, or disabled people remain in bed for many unnecessary days, weeks, and even months.

Prolonged bedrest has many negative effects on people and their families. Some of these negative effects include:

• Shallow breathing, which can lead to pneumonia.

• Decreased circulation, leading to muscle spasms and decubitus ulcers (bedsores).

• Contracture, or tightening of muscles, which makes bathing, dressing, and transfers difficult.

• Shrinking of muscle bulk from inactivity.

• Altered balance and tolerance for standing upright.

• Light or restless sleeping patterns.

• Decreased appetite.

• Constipation.

• Altered self concept; feelings of hopelessness.

• Decreased interpersonal and social interactions.

• Inability to participate in 'normal' activities.

Overall, being confined to a bed or even confined to the home because of a lack of knowledge about transfers severely restricts the person and their caregiver from engaging in everyday activities which are very important to general well-being and quality of life.

Before we elaborate on the several different types of transfers, we would like to clarify some general myths about people's ability to safely transfer a person.

A common myth is that 'the person doing the transfer must be physically strong and tall in order to transfer a person. If you have a bad back, arthritis, other medical conditions, or are over the age of 50, you should never attempt any kind of transfer at all.' First, we would like to point out that although physical strength, height, and weight do have their advantages, they are not essential to perform a safe and effective transfer. Secondly, a bad back, other medical condition, or advancing age *do not* in themselves always restrict a person from doing a transfer.

Performing safe transfers depends primarily upon being trained by a qualified professional in the appropriate transfer technique for your situation. Physical and occupational therapists are the specialists you would best consult to obtain this information. Be certain that one or the other of these professionals have trained you before you attempt any transfer. These professionals will consider and assess not only the person to be transferred, but also your physical capabilities, medical history, or other information which would impact on your ability to perform a transfer.

Never perform any transfer until you have been professionally trained and tested and have consulted with your physician. If this was not done while the family member was in the hospital, call your local Visiting Nurse Association or home health care agency and request training by a licensed physical or occupational therapist. The health and safety of both of you are extremely important, and are not to be taken lightly.

The transfer procedures that are outlined in this chapter are to serve as general guidelines and reminders only, and are not intended to substitute for actual professional training by a physical or occupational therapist. As each person and caregiver are different, so too are specific transfer instructions.

Basic transfer procedures will be presented in this chapter. Each one in turn will always follow the first eight steps. Individual procedures will therefore begin with Step Nine.

Step 1

Explain the entire procedure to the person before you begin, so that they will know what to expect and how they can help you.

Step 2

Prepare the environment for the transfer. Make sure that the immediate area is safe: remove throw rugs, extension cords, over-the-bed tables, waste baskets, or any other items which may interfere with safety.

Step 3

Raise the bed until the person's waist is level with your waist. Depending on your height, the person's feet may or may not touch the floor.

Step 4

Prepare the person for the transfer:

A. Pull back the bed covers and fold them neatly at the end of the bed. Make certain that the person's feet are clear from any bed covers. Assist the person in dressing appropriately for their modesty, comfort, and the particular occasion.

B. Lock the wheels on the bed.

C. Remove the bed rail on the side that you are going to do the transfer and put it under the bed out of your way.

D. If the person is using oxygen, make sure that the tubing is long enough to reach to wherever you are transferring the person. Or, if the tubing is too long, drape it out of the way so it is not tripped over. If the person has a catheter, detach the urine collection bag from the bed and hook it onto your own belt loop or pocket. Check to be sure that the catheter and connecting tubing are not tangled or caught in any clothing. Also make certain that there is sufficient tubing to reach to where you are transferring the person.

Step 5

If the person is able, have them scoot up to the head of the bed, as discussed in Chapter Six (pages 67-68). If the person is unable to do so independently, assist them as shown below.

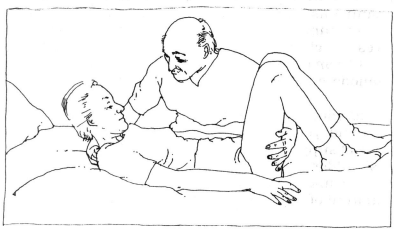

Step 6

Raise the head of the bed as high as possible. The closer the person is to a full sitting position, the easier the transfer will be. If the person is uncomfortable in a full sitting position, raise the head of the bed to the position at which they will be comfortable. Again check oxygen and catheter tubing.

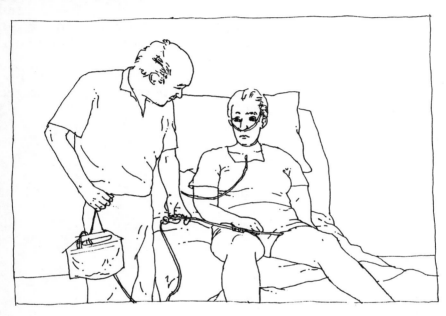

Step 7

Prepare yourself for the transfer. Use only the least intrusive assistance as is necessary, and encourage the person to use an overhead trapeze or his or her own arm muscles to push themselves upright in bed. If the person does not get out of bed often, allow them to sit for three to five minutes in order for them to accommodate to an upright posture.

Remind yourself of the person's degree of need for assistance. Remind yourself of your own limitations. Maintain a broad base of support by standing with your feet apart (as wide as your shoulders), knees flexed to bring you at eye level with the person, trunk and head in an upright position, and one foot slightly in front of the other. If you are wearing trousers, slacks, or other snug fitting clothing, hike them over your knees so that you'll be able to bend with ease. Keep in mind that you will be maintaining your center of gravity by remaining in close physical proximity to the person, and that you will be lifting with your legs, not your back. You should be aware that the first few times you do a transfer your calf muscles will be sore, because you are lifting completely with your legs, and not at all with your back. When doing a correct transfer you will never feel a strain or pull on your back. Never lift the person under the arm pits or pull them by the arms. These methods may result in serious nerve damage or dislocation of the shoulder.

The following illustrations show the correct and incorrect bed height for safe and easy transfers.

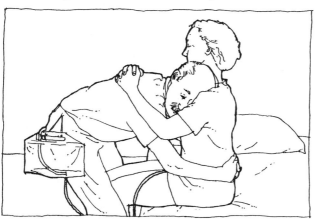

Incorrect

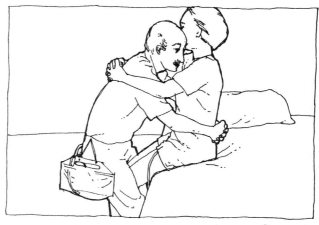

Correct

Transfer Belts

The transfers in this chapter are shown without the use of transfer belts (gait belts, walking belts). A transfer belt is a five inch wide belt made of heavy cotton with a buckle closure. It has three loop handles – one on each side and one on the back. This belt is worn around the waist of the person that is going to be transferred or walked. The person doing the transfer puts one or both hands through various handles to transfer the person and/or to help balance while walking.

Although transfer belts are recommended by some professionals, we do not recommend them for the average transfer in home care.

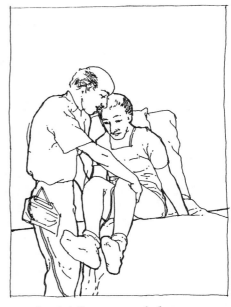

Assist the person's knees over the side of the bed.

Step 8

Have the necessary equipment ready – cane, walker, wheelchair, or commode at the side of the bed. Then assist the person in coming to a sitting position on the side of the bed, as depicted to the right:

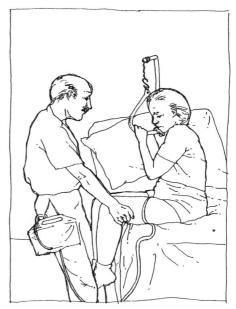

Have the person scoot, or gently pull them, to the edge of the bed.

Specific Transfers

Bed to standing with use of cane or walker.

Step 9

Hand cane to person or position the walker at a 60 degree angle to the side of the person. Place one or two hands as needed around the person's back, approximately in the region just below their shoulder blades (scapulae) or slightly lower, whichever feels most comfortable and secure to you.

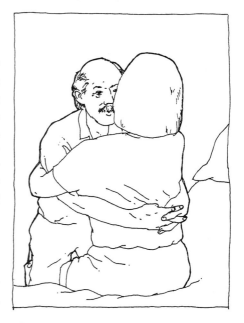

Step 10

Tell the person that on the count of three, you will both stand up together. Double check the position of your feet so that they are positioned around the person's feet to allow your legs to provide support for the person's legs.

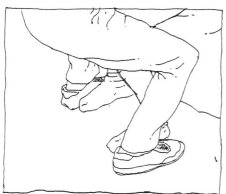

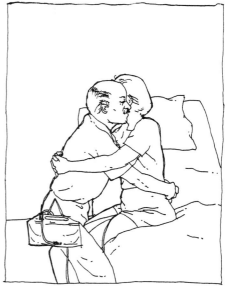

If the person has good strength in their arms, tell them to push up from the bed or chair with their arms, and not to pull themselves up by grabbing the walker (as it will not be steady enough to support their weight pulling on it).

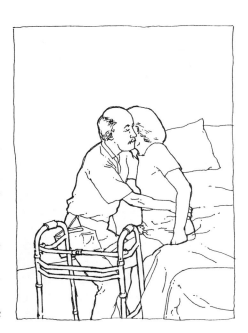

When a person has one weak side, as with a stroke, they should always be transferred to their strongest side, and the weaker side should be supported.

Instruct the person to lean forward while standing – this will assist both of you to maintain a common center of gravity. Many people are afraid of falling and frequently lean backwards. This makes the transfer difficult and dangerous.

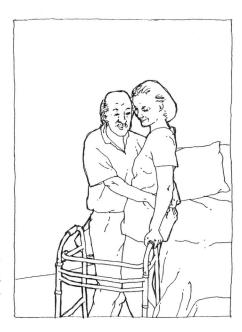

Step 11

On the count of three, straighten your knees and provide the necessary physical assistance by guiding the person up with your hands.

Remember not to lift up with your back. As the person comes close to an erect posture, have them hold onto the walker or cane for support as you prepare to remove your physical guidance.

Step 12

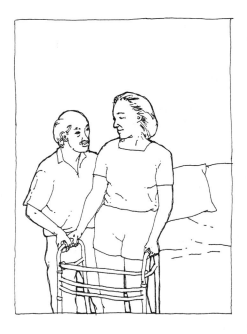

Further assist the person into a fully erect standing posture. Before you remove your hands from the person, ask them if they are ready for you to let go.

Assess their balance and strength for independent standing by observing and feeling their degree of steadiness. Release your physical assistance when they are ready to stand on their own.

Dependent stand-pivot transfer to wheelchair or commode.

Step 9

A. Wheelchair. Bring the wheelchair to the side of the bed and place it at a 60 degree angle. **Put on both brakes**, remove both foot rests and the arm rest on the side nearest the bed.

Note: If you have a family member who needs any assistance in transferring from the bed to a wheelchair, be certain that the wheelchair has removable foot rests and arm rests. *Never* transfer a person into a wheelchair that has fixed foot and arm rests. Should you have this type of wheelchair in your home, please contact the agency or durable medical supply company from whom you obtained the wheelchair and have it exchanged.

A wheelchair with removable foot and arm rests will be more expensive to rent or purchase, but the additional expense will prevent the possibility of serious injury to you and your family member.

B. Commode. As with the wheelchair, place it at the side of the bed at a 60 degree angle. Because commodes do not have wheels, they also do not have brakes to secure them from moving. Therefore be certain that all telescoping legs are the same height and that they are all firmly and securely placed on the floor.

Some commodes have arm rests that either remove or drop to the side. If you have one of these commodes, either remove or drop the arm rest on the side nearest the bed.

The illustrations on the top of the next page show the proper positioning of the wheelchair and commode.

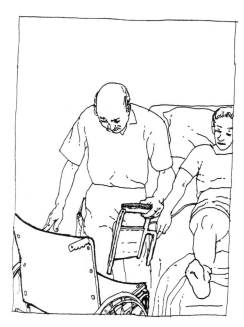

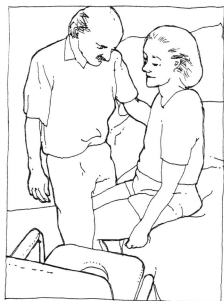

Step 10

Firmly stabilize the person's knees by placing your knees on the sides of the person's knees.

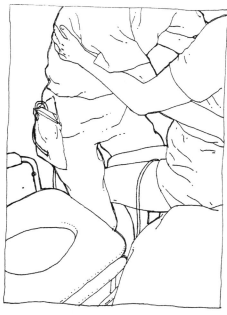

Step 11

Assist the person in lean-
ing forward, over their knees,
and scooting up to the edge of
the bed. It helps some persons
to remember by telling them to
'keep their nose over their toes.'
Place your hands around the
middle of the person's back, or
down closer to the buttocks if it
affords you more stability.

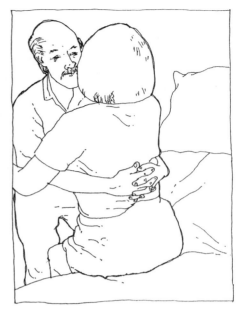

Step 12

Gently rock back and forth
with the person to gain momentum, and on the count of
three, straighten out your knees
and hips, taking care not to lift
with your back. As you raise
up, stabilize the person's feet
and knees with your own.

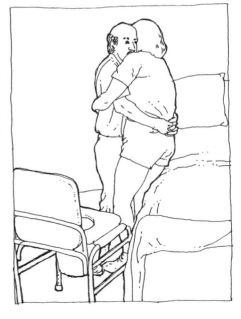

Step 13

At this point, either come to a full standing position with the person and prepare yourself to pivot with your legs after you have stabilized yourself and the person (shown below). . .

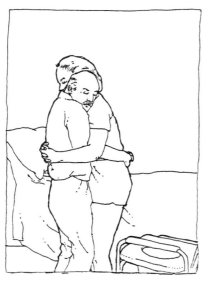 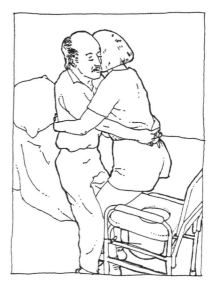

. . . or use your momentum to pivot the person immediately onto the other surface while the person is in a semi-seated position (shown below).

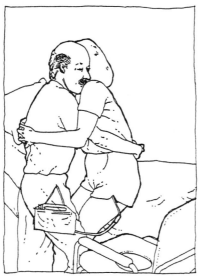 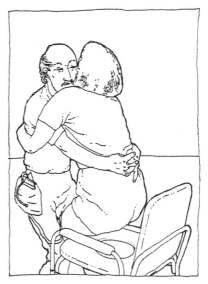

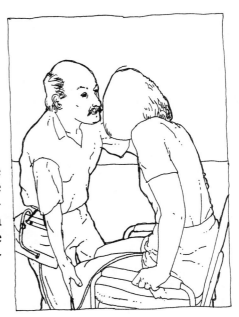

Step 14

Secure the person on the new transfer surface before releasing your physical assistance. For example, have them scoot back onto the commode or wheelchair for maximal postural support.

When returning (transferring) the person to bed from a wheelchair . . .

A. Lower the bed to its lowest position.

B. Lower the head of the bed so that the bed is completely flat.

C. Bring the wheelchair close to the head of the bed so that when you stand and pivot the person, their buttocks will arrive at the point where the head of the bed attaches to the bed. In this manner, when the person is back in bed, you will not have to pull them up.

Transfers Using a Sliding Board

If the person has very weak legs which are unable to bear much or any weight at all, your therapist may show you how the person can transfer with a sliding board. A sliding board is a small rectangular piece of wood or plastic material (30 inches long and 8-9 inches wide) that acts as a 'bridge' between the two transfer surfaces. The person is able to 'slide' across this 'bridge' to go from one location to another.

The basic steps for sliding board transfers are slightly different than other transfers.

Step 1:

Equalize the level of the two surfaces as much as possible.

This may mean that you have to raise or lower the bed, commode, or chair. Consider that it will be difficult for the person to 'slide' if they have to go uphill.

Step 2:

Prepare the environment, as outlined on page 105, Step 2.

Step 3:

Prepare the person, as outlined on page 106, Step 4.

Step 4:

Assist the person into a sitting position on the side of the bed, as outlined on page 109, Step 8.

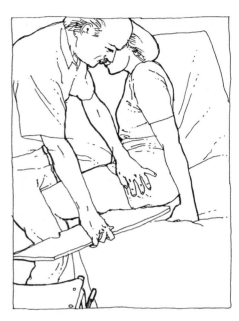

Step 5:

Put one end of the sliding board underneath the person's buttocks, and place the other end securely onto the surface being transferred to. If you are transferring to a wheelchair, be sure to remove the foot rests and the arm rest nearest the bed.

Step 6:

Encourage the person to push up with their arms extended to begin sliding along the board. Give whatever physical assistance is necessary. Always provide contact support to make sure that the person does not fall off of the board. Check to make sure that the board is secure on both surfaces. Be sure that the person's fingers are not under the sliding board during the transfer, to avoid pinching when the person slides along the board.

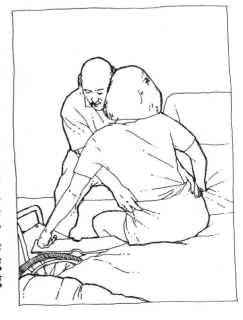

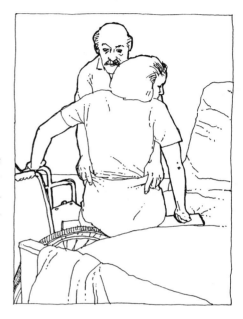

Step 7:

Guide the person along the board and onto the other surface, always encouraging them to push themselves along with their arms extended.

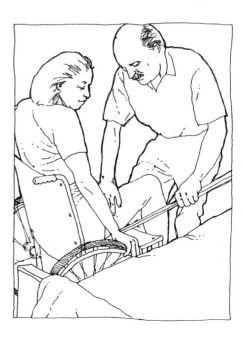

Step 8:

When the person is securely seated in the new area, remove the board from underneath the person's buttocks. Replace the foot and arm rests.

Transfers In and Out of Automobiles

There are two basic wheelchair to car transfers: stand pivot and sliding board. The stand pivot transfer is used when the person can use their legs to help with the transfer. The sliding board transfer is used when the person cannot use their legs to assist in the transfer. Whichever transfer you use, do not attempt it with a car until you have mastered the regular stand pivot or sliding board transfer as outlined earlier in this chapter.

Before you plan any car outing, obtain a handicapped parking permit, even if the person is only going to be using a wheelchair for a short period of time. A handicapped parking permit bestows two great advantages: a parking space close to the building that you are going to enter and an extra wide space between cars to maneuver the wheelchair.

Stand pivot transfer

Step 1:

Park your car where there is ample room on the passenger side to open the door to its fullest extent. There should be enough room to maneuver the wheelchair, and the ground should be level and solid for safe footing.

Step 2:

Open the front seat passenger door as wide as it will go, and put the passenger seat back as far as it will go.

Step 3:

Standing in front of the person, pull the wheelchair towards you to about two feet from the seat of the car. The angle, about 60 degrees, depends upon how wide the car door opens.

Step 4:

Remove both foot rests and put them out of the way. Pull the wheelchair as close to the car as possible while at the same time leaving just enough room for yourself and the person to stand and pivot. **Lock both wheels.**

Reverse both arm rests. This puts the arm rests at the front of the chair and provides the person with a place to put their hands. This helps the person scoot themself to the front of the wheelchair as well as assist themself in coming to a standing position.

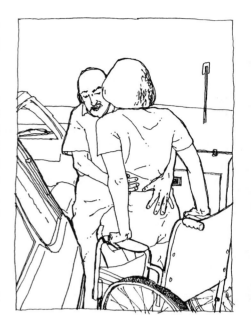

Step 5:

As with the standing pivot transfer described previously, assist the person to a standing position.

Step 6:

If the person can use one or both arms, have them find a comfortable position to place their hands (the roof of the car and/or the door window frame. This will allow them a few seconds to secure their balance before you pivot them.

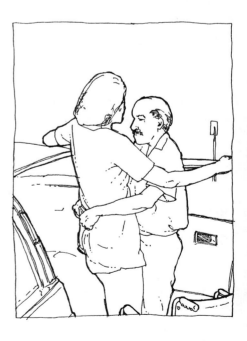

Step 7:

Assist the person in backing up until their legs are touching the side of the car.

Step 8:

Have the person put one or both arms inside the car (on the back seat and/or on the dashboard) to stabilize them.

Step 9:

Assist the person in squatting down to sit on the side of the seat. While you are doing this, keep one of your hands around the person's waist, and the other hand on top of their head to prevent it from hitting the top of the car.

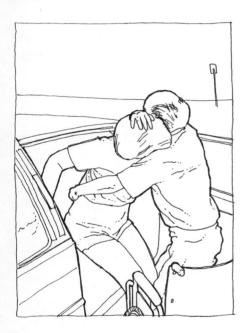 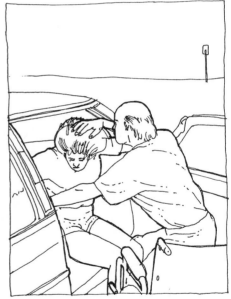

Step 10:

Remove both arm rests. Put both foot and arm rests in the car. Leaving the wheels locked, fold the wheelchair, and put it in the car. Depending on the size of your car, you can either put it on the seat, on the floor of the back seat, or in the trunk.

Reverse this procedure for transferring the person from the car back to the wheelchair. When you reach your destination be certain that you park your car in either a handicapped parking spot or a parking spot where no other car can park next to the passenger side of the car. If you park in a regular parking spot where there is an empty parking spot next to the passenger side, the chances of you returning to your car and finding a car parked next to yours is just about 100%. Should this happen, there will not be enough room for you to either open your car door fully or maneuver the wheelchair.

Sliding board transfer

Step 1:

Make certain you have a sliding board that is 30 inches long and 8-9 inches wide. Park your car where there is ample room on the passenger side to maneuver the wheelchair.

Step 2:

Open the front seat passenger door as wide as it will go, and put the passenger seat back as far as it will go.

Step 3:

Remove both foot rests and the arm rest nearest the side of the car. Standing in front of the person, pull the wheelchair towards you to about two feet from the seat of the car, or just close enough to move behind the wheelchair.

Step 4:

Go behind the wheelchair. Have the person hold their legs up so their feet are just off the ground. Push the wheelchair firmly up against the car as far as it will go and **lock both wheels**.

Step 5:

Have the person lean to their right so that you can slip the sliding board under their left buttock (see sliding board transfers pages 118 to 120).

Step 6:

Make certain that the sliding board is placed so that enough of it is under the left buttocks and bridges sufficiently into the car seat. Note that since the height of the wheelchair is likely to be higher than the car seat, the portion of the sliding board that extends into the car may not rest evenly on the car seat. This is okay. When the person begins to move across the transfer board, it will slowly and safely tilt until it rests firmly on the car seat.

Step 7:

When the sliding board is in place, assist the person in putting their legs into the car. Both feet should be firmly placed on the floor of the car.

Step 8:

Have the person place their right hand on the right arm rest and their left hand on the transfer board. Then place your hands on the person's waist. (*Not* under the arm pits!)

Step 9:

On the count of three, assist the person in sliding with three or four movements across the transfer board until they are in the center of the passenger seat. If the person is unable to reach the center of the passenger seat, go to the driver's side of the car. Get into the driver's seat on your knees. Put one hand under the person's knees and the other hand around their waist. Gently pull them to the center of the seat.

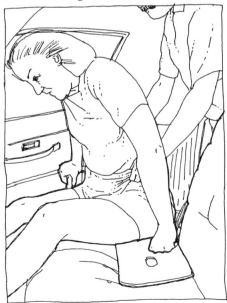

Step 10:

Return to the passenger side of the car if you went to the driver's side. Pull the sliding board out from under the person, secure the seat belt, lock and close the door, and put the wheelchair into the car (see step 10 of the stand pivot transfer procedure from wheelchair to car, page 123).

When you reach your destination be certain that you park your car in either a handicapped parking spot or a parking spot where no other car can park next to the passenger side of the car. If you park in a regular parking spot where there is an empty parking spot next to the passenger side, the chances of you returning to your car and finding a car parked next to yours is just about 100%. Should this happen, there will not be enough room for you to either open your car door fully or maneuver the wheelchair.

These examples are just general guidelines for some very common and basic transfer procedures. Remember to consult your physical or occupational therapist for very specific instruction and training in these techniques, or others, if they are warranted.

With practice and perseverance, you will be able to help the person get up, about, moving, and participating in the world once again. Simple mobility between bed and wheelchair, wheelchair and toilet, or wheelchair and car will open up a whole new set of opportunities and experiences, leading back into normal participation in everyday activities once again.

8

Accessing Home Health Care and Community Resources

Once you have a sense that you have a need for some assistance in caring for an ill or disabled person at home, what do you do then? How do you determine exactly what type of agency to call upon? How do you find them? How will they be paid? How can you assure yourself that the person is qualified and reliable? There is no easy answer to any of these questions, but a few guidelines may help.

First of all, will you need a health care professional, such as a registered nurse or a therapist, to render the care? If so, you likely will want to call upon a certified home health agency, or in certain states such as New York State, possibly a long term home health care program if the person's needs are long term in nature and Medicaid reimbursement is available. In many communities, home health agencies are operated by visiting nursing associations. Sometimes they are sponsored by your local health department; many hospitals have home care departments. Being "certified" means that the agencies meet stringent guidelines set up by the federal government, and because they demonstrate compliance with these guidelines, they are permitted to bill Medicare and Medicaid directly for their services. They provide skilled care, usually rehabilitation oriented, to deal with an acute or unstable condition, and for a relatively short period of time. Often these professionals teach the person and/or families how to provide the care themselves.

If the need is more for help with activities of daily living, such as bathing, dressing, meal preparation, and light house-keeping, a homemaker agency, or proprietary home care agency will be able to provide a worker that is usually paid by the person on an hourly basis. In certain states, these agencies are required to be licensed by the state's health department. Asking about licensure is one way that a person can determine whether or not the agency meets basic guidelines about screening their employees, making sure they have adequate training, and are properly supervised.

If the person in need of care has a terminal illness (about six months or less to live), a hospice may be appropriate. Hospice caregivers not only provide direct hands-on profes-sional care, but also provide for a holistic approach to emotional and spiritual needs of the dying and their families as well. Hospices provide home care, and often some very short-term in-patient care at a hospital or free-standing facility to stabilize the medical condition of the person, or to give the family caregivers a short respite from care. Hospices are also "certified" and can be reimbursed by Medicaid and Medicare. It should be kept in mind that whenever care is billed to Medicare or any other third party insurance, a doctor's order for the care is required.

To locate the appropriate caregiver, there are certain key agencies available in most communities that can be contacted and that will be able to direct you to one or more sources of the help you need.

If the person is elderly, try contacting the local department of senior services or office for aging for information about services available in your community for seniors. The depart-ment of social services may also provide information about care available, especially if the person has a low income. The social work department or discharge planning staff at your local hospital(s) also are a good source of information because it is their job to link people up with appropriate home care services when they are needed immediately following a hospitalization.

Other likely sources of information may be organizations such as Catholic Charities, Jewish Family Services, Episcopal

Charities, the Salvation Army, or the United Way office. Your physician may have knowledge about home care services — some more than others make it their business to become familiar with home care resources. It can't hurt to try them, especially when a doctor's order may be required for you to seek third party reimbursement for the care.

The yellow pages of the phone book is another way to find which agencies operate in your community. However, if the agency is not certified or licensed, here are a few questions you should ask to assure yourself you will be receiving good help:

1. Do the employees have to complete a training program? How long is it and what does it consist of?

2. Who supervises the employees? What are their qualifications? How often does the supervisor oversee the care right at the home?

3. Can you contact the agency at any time of any day, or are supervisory staff only available during business hours?

4. Are the staff bonded and does the agency carry liability insurance?

5. What recourse do you have if the worker provided doesn't show up, or provides unsatisfactory care?

6. How much will you have to pay and how will billing be handled?

Apart from the extent of medical and personal care your family member may require, please do not forget, overlook, or underestimate, the importance of providing social, leisure, recreational opportunities as they are vital to quality of living.

Transportation

If you are going to use your own car, the first thing you need to do is to apply for a handicapped parking permit. This is done by calling or stopping into your local police precinct/mayor's office of services for the handicapped and obtain an application. This application has sections to be filled out by you and your physician. These applications are generally processed quickly. In about a week you will receive a parking permit card that you place on the dashboard on the driver's side of the car. This card can be removed and placed in any vehicle the person will be traveling in. This special parking permit will allow you to park very close to your destination — saving you and your family member literally thousands of steps and countless energy.

If you do not have access to a car, outings into the community will be a bit more difficult to arrange. Is there a neighbor that would be willing to provide transportation? Can your synagogue or church arrange regular or periodic transportation?

These days most larger communities have agencies that provide transportation. Contact your community center, or your municipality transportation center. Buses and subways often have accommodations for people in wheelchairs. In many cities people in wheelchairs can travel free. If you are traveling out of town by train and/or plane, tell your ticket agent, or travel agent, you will be traveling with a person in a wheelchair. You will be surprised with the special accommodations that are provided. Also, when making hotel or motel accommodations, ask them what services they provide.

If you plan to go to the movies, a play, concert, or to a sporting event, call the ticket office and ask what they provide. These calls will save you much frustration and allow for a pleasant outing for all involved.

Being home over long periods of time can become tiring and frustrating for the caregiver as well as the person. No matter how caring and loving everyone is, people need a break — time to be alone and to do their own thing, or just to have some time to catch up on personal and/or family needs. Some long term home health care programs, nursing homes and hospices provide respite services. These services provide a place where your family member can spend a weekend or a week, while you simply rest and catch up on your work, or go out of town for a family gathering or vacation.

Many churches, synagogues, city and/or county organizations provide social day care programs and/or senior citizen programs. They provide a wide range of services which can include lunch, opportunities to meet and socialize with others, recreational/craft programs, and sometimes transportation. Community centers are well known for their excellent programs and services. Check also with your county or city parks and recreational departments.

If your family member is in need of constant or periodic oxygen, call your supplier and ask for portable travel tanks. These tanks are small and lightweight. They can be hung over the back of a wheelchair or carried over your shoulder. With a portable oxygen tank you can take your family member out into the backyard, around the block, to parties, etc.

As a general rule, a greater variety of help from multiple sources is available in a large metropolitan area, and more scarce in a rural area. However, in the country, often neighbors are more accustomed to helping one another out and can be an informal source of assistance. One of the secrets in obtaining the help you need is simply to ask, and keep asking. Ask the sources cited above, ask health care professionals you know, and if you are lucky enough to have a formal information and referral resource in your community, ask there. Home health care is rapidly expanding at the present time and that can only be good news for those who are in need of it.

If you, and/or your family member has multiple sclerosis, muscular dystrophy, Alzheimer's, has had a stroke, is blind or partially sighted, look in your yellow pages for the appropriate association (Also see Appendix A). These agencies have excellent services, information and programs for you and/or your family member. Please don't hesitate to call or write to them. Explain your situation and needs. If you or your family member is or has ever been a member of the Rotary, Lions, Kiwanis, or any other like organization, contact them. Even if they may not have direct services, they may be able to direct you to needed services.

The American Association of Retired People (AARP) is an excellent organization. They can provide you with valuable information through their magazine, *Modern Maturity*.

There are a lot of caring and concerned organizations in your community that can provide invaluable support and services. I know you may be overwhelmed with your situation and not feel that you have the time or energy to cope with organizing social, leisure, or recreational activities for your family member. Please be assured that both of you need them. First, start by asking your family member what they would like to do. Initially they may say, "Nothing." This response is not uncommon. When one has not felt well and/or has lost functional ability, one loses interests and home and bed become a safe place to retreat. Nevertheless, keep encouraging them. Remind them that they and you need a break from each other and that by getting out they can meet people and do enjoyable things. As such you will both benefit, if by nothing more than having something new to talk about instead of aches and pains and misery.

9

When Home Care Is No Longer Possible

There were days, before hospitals were available in most communities, where the sole source of health care was a country doctor who made his rounds with black bag in hand and with a heart full of dedication and regard for his patients. As the population grew and larger communities were formed, a larger supply of doctors became available, and health care became more structured and organized as modern hospitals and convalescent homes were founded.

Medicine became more sophisticated as scientific knowledge grew. Replacing the doctor's black bag was the CT scanner, the IV pumps, and the respirators. Many people believed that care of ill family members could no longer be placed in the hands of a loving family simply because modern medicine had become so complex. The entire concept of home care was lost as large institutions were constructed and staffed in order to service many patients who shared similar medical difficulties.

Today there is a re-emphasis on home care due to the rising costs of prolonged hospital stays. Doctors are now discharging patients who may still be acutely ill, but who have potential to be cared for in the home setting. This adds a significantly greater share of responsibility on family caregivers who are now called upon to manage the medical care of patients during acute phases of illness.

Unfortunately, there are no rules or guidelines for family members to follow in regard to what they can realistically manage in caring for a loved one at home. There are, however, key issues to consider which can help in determining how practical home care may be in any individual case. Under no situation should a family feel that they are "forced" to provide home care for someone, as it is often not feasible due to many intervening factors.

One cardinal principle for all families to remember is that the care they provide can only be as functional as the family itself is. In other words, if the family is chaotic, disorganized, divided, and confused, all this will be reflected back in the care that they will be able to provide. As the old saying goes, you can't get organized in a disorganized environment.

Sick people require great attention: it is very difficult to provide and manage home care unless there is a well-developed support system in place. This support system has to include family members, friends, home care providers, medical equipment, vendors, and hospital discharge planners. Sometimes, despite all efforts and good intentions of the hospital discharge planners, home placement becomes riddled with difficulties. Lack of available home care services, geographic isolation in rural areas, lack of money to pay for home health aides or medical equipment, poor health of other family members, complexity of providing medical care, and a myriad of other problems may interfere with the "optimal" discharge plan. Family members must be realistic and honest about the resources they have available to them and what they can reasonably expect to provide. There are times, despite all good plans and attempts to organize a workable home care plan, the pieces of the plan just can't seem to fit together.

One family rallied together when their mother was discharged from the hospital following a stroke. The children alternately spent the evenings and nights sleeping at the parent's home while home health aides cared for the mother during the day when she did not attend a medical day treatment program in the community. Even the woman's husband, himself limited by weakness and chest pain caused by a severe heart attack, learned to test blood sugars and administer insulin to his diabetic spouse. The visiting physical therapist taught the woman how to walk with the use of a walker, and gave her exercises for her weak arm. The visiting occupational therapist helped the family acquire equipment so that the woman could take a bath in the bathtub, get in and out of the wheelchair van safely, and taught her ways to still be able to participate in cooking the family dinners as she did prior to her stroke. Even this seemingly "perfect" plan had its rough edges: the husband began experiencing chest pains and had to curtail his activities, the children's families were strained as time and money were spent in caring for the ill parents, there were days when the home health aides did not show up for work, and the woman's diabetes fluctuated drastically, which at times affected her level of alertness and ability to participate in her own care. Home care was just not working out.

There may come a time when a family has exhausted all of the community resources, when there is no more energy or strength to rally everyone together, and when no one's needs are being met in the home environment. It is at this point in time that options beyond home care must be investigated.

Often, the most difficult part of home care is knowing when to say, "This is too much for me. I just can't do this anymore." The family may often feel guilty that they were unable to continually provide for the ill family member in the home. The family must come to understand that not all situations are functional for home care. It is very difficult to care for a loved one who has had a stroke and is unable to dress, bathe, or walk. It is very difficult to care for a loved one with any debilitating condition, especially a condition requiring stoma care, decubitus care, and so on. No one invites the prospect of hospitalization, an adult domiciliary, or a nursing home, but for many families these are the only alternatives.

As family members who may feel overburdened and unable to provide care anymore, you are likely to experience feelings of anxiety and guilt and even perhaps failure. It is at this time that you need to step back from the situation and breathe deeply. Just because things do not work out as you may have planned, it is not necessarily anyone's "fault." Carrying this "no-fault" attitude with you as you investigate the possibility of nursing home placement will help you tremendously in maintaining a realistically positive and understanding approach to this difficult decision.

Do not approach this decision alone. If at all possible, include the ill family member in the decision. At a time when they have lost so much control over their lives, offering them this respect and consideration may be the most important gift you could ever give them. If they are unable to functionally be a part of the decision or if they are unable to be rationale and realistic, make your plans carefully without them; be kind and firm when it is time to explain that this is your last and only choice.

Talk to your priest, minister, rabbi, or counselor. Undoubtedly, these people have been approached with this difficulty before. Tell them about how hard you tried to make home care work, and tell them about your hesitations and fears. These people may help you immeasurably: they will help you and your family cope with this situation, and they may also be able to suggest nursing homes where they frequent and provide services.

Call up the hospital discharge planner or the director of patient services of your home health care agency. These people are very knowledgeable of "the system." They know the ins and outs, what paperwork is required, who you can talk to about financial assistance or legal advocacy. It is likely that they know the social workers and admission coordinators in the local nursing homes as they work with them on a daily basis. They can help you communicate with and coordinate placement with the assistance of the doctor. They can give you a list of nursing homes in the area, and they can advise you if there is a waiting list for any of these facilities.

Visit the nursing homes. This may take time to go to each facility, but is essential in choosing what will be the best new home for the ill family member. Be critical as you ask the following questions:

1. Is it certified and licensed by the state?

2. Do they have a record of state survey results for you to examine?

3. Is it well kept and clean?

4. Is it nicely decorated?

5. What percentage of the residents are restrained (physically or chemically)?

6. What percentage of the residents developed muscle contractures?

7. Is it staffed by employees or agency fill-ins?

8. What is the staff to patient ratio?

9. What is the neighborhood like?

10. What do the people who live there think of it?

11. How do their families feel about the facility?

12. Are there private or semi-private rooms?

13. Ask what services are available: do they offer occupational, physical, and speech therapy?

14. Do residents dine in their rooms or in a congregate/family style?

15. What is the activities department like: do they cater to the patients who require more care as well as those who require less care?

16. Are there activities offered on the weekends and during the evenings?

17. Are families regularly included in the plan of care?

18. Do they encourage and request family attendance at resident care conferences?

19. How will all these services be paid for?

20. Does the nursing home help you deal with any financial concerns?

Talk to the residents who live there. Talk with their families. Talk to the staff. Do the residents and staff have pride in the facility? As you tour the facility, does your guide greet the residents cheerfully and by name? Do the residents respond in acknowledgment? Does your guide stop to pick up a piece of paper off of the floor or stop to tell a nurse that a patient requested to be toileted? These will all be clues to you which will help distinguish the facilities where there is a clear sense of pride and love for the residents and a concern for the quality of care that is provided.

No list of questions can ever be comprehensive. Think of your own specific concerns. Don't be afraid to ask questions or to challenge. Long term care is a booming business and these nursing homes compete with each other. If you are not satisfied with the answers you are given, continue to shop elsewhere. Be a conscientious health care consumer.

No nursing home is flawless. Staffing may never be perfect, personal effects may be misplaced and lost, residents may have to wait their turn to be toileted as nursing aides respond to another resident's needs. Still, you will be able to distinguish those homes where these are chronic problems of ill-management as opposed to when these problems are infrequent and quickly ameliorated by a hard working and dedicated staff.

Again, remember that just because home care didn't work, it is not necessarily someone's "fault." Maintain a positive attitude, shop carefully, and above all remain highly sensitive, respectful, and honest with each other. This is the time when you need to understand and support each other most.

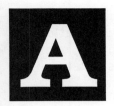

HealthFinder

Federal Health Information Clearinghouse*

National AIDS Information Clearinghouse (NAIC)
P.O. Box 6003, Rockville, MD 20850; (800) 458-5231.

Responds to the needs of health professionals involved in the development and delivery of AIDS programs; ensures that the general public has access to information on AIDS; provides technical assistance to organizations involved in the fight against AIDS, particularly state health departments; assists in the development and assessment of resources; supports all AIDS information delivery services of the Centers for Disease Control, including the National AIDS hotline (800-342-AIDS; 800-344-SIDA-Spanish); and distributes single copies of selected publications. NAIC Resource Center open to the public by appointment from 9 a.m. to 5 p.m., Monday through Friday.

National Clearinghouse for ALCOHOL and Drug Information (NCADI)
P.O. Box 2345, Rockville, MD 20852; (301) 468-2600.

Gathers and disseminates current knowledge on alcohol and drug-related subjects. Services include subject searches on an in-house automated database and responses to inquires for statistics and other information. Develops resource materials and operates the Regional Alcohol and Drug Awareness Resource (RADAR), a nationwide linkage of drug information

* Reprinted by permission. National Health Information Center.

centers. Library available and open to the public Monday through Friday, 9:30 a.m. to 4:30 p.m. Contains information on all aspects of alcohol and other drug abuse including over 80 journals, newsletters, and major U.S. newspapers. Distributes a variety of publications on alcohol and drug abuse.

ALZHEIMER'S DISEASE Education and Referral Center
8737 Colesville Road, Silver Spring, MD 20910; (301) 495-3311.

Sponsored by the National Institute on Aging. Provides information on Alzheimer's disease of special interest to health and service professionals, patients and their families, caregivers, and the general public. Publications available on Alzheimer's disease and self-help groups.

National ARTHRITIS and Musculoskeletal and Skin Disease Information Clearinghouse (NAMSIC)
P.O. Box AMS, Bethesda, MD 20892; (301) 468-3235.

Identifies print and audiovisual educational materials concerning arthritis and musculoskeletal diseases, and serves as an information exchange for individuals and organizations involved in public, professional, and patient education. Requests are answered by searching the clearinghouse's database and other bibliographic sources and by making referrals to appropriate resources. Distributes a variety of publications for professionals on topics related to arthritis and musculoskeletal and skin diseases.

National AUDIOVISUAL Center (NAC)
National Archives and Records Administration, 8700 Edgeworth, Drive, Capitol Heights, MD 20743-3701; (301) 763-1896 in Metropolitan Washington, DC., (301) 763-6025 (fax), (800) 638-1300.

Provides a central source for purchasing or renting more than 8,000 federally produced audiovisual programs available to the public. Catalogues and referrals to free loan sources are provided at no cost. Several catalogues cover health-related topics, including alcohol and drug abuse, dentistry, emergency medical services, industrial safety, medicine, and nursing.

National Library Service for the BLIND and Physically Handicapped (NLS)

Library of Congress, 1291 Taylor Street NW., Washington, DC 20542; (202) 707-9287, (800) 424-8567.

Consists of a network of 56 regional and over 100 local libraries working in cooperation with the Library of Congress to provide free library service to anyone who is unable to read or use standard printed materials because of visual or physical impairment. Delivers books and magazine in recorded form or in Braille to eligible readers by postage-free mail and provides postage for their return. Specially designed phonographs and cassette players are also loaned free to persons borrowing "talking books." Provides information on blindness, physical handicaps, and library services to special groups on request. A list of participating local and regional libraries is available.

CANCER Information Service (CIS)

Office of Cancer Communications, National Cancer Institute, Building 31, Room 10A24, 9000 Rockville Pike, Bethesda, MD 20892; (800) 4-CANCER, (301) 496-8664 (project officer).

Provides information about cancer and cancer-related resources to the general public and to cancer patients and their families. Callers are automatically put in touch with the CIS office serving their area. Inquiries are handled by health educators and trained volunteers. Spanish-speaking staff members are available during daytime hours to callers from the following areas: California, Florida, Georgia, Illinois, northern New Jersey, New York, and Texas. Distributes free publications of the National Cancer Institute.

National DIABETES INFORMATION Clearinghouse (NDIC)

Box NDIC, Bethesda, MD 20892; (301) 468-2162.

Collects and disseminates information about patient education materials. Maintains a meeting registry that includes regional, national, and international meetings, congresses, and symposia of interest to the diabetes community. Distributes its own publications, as well as other diabetes related materials. Library collection of approximately 5,000 items is open to the public, although materials do not circulate. Maintains an automated database of patient and professional materials.

National DIGESTIVE DISEASES Information Clearinghouse (NDDIC)

P.O. Box NDDIC, Bethesda, MD 20892; (301) 468-6344.

Provides a central information resource on digestive health and the prevention and management of digestive diseases. Develops, identifies, and distributes educational materials; encourages production of needed materials; and responds to requests for information. Maintains an automated database of patient education materials.

Clearinghouse on DISABILITY INFORMATION

Office of Special Education and Rehabilitative Services, Switzer Building, Room 3132, 330 C Street SW., Washington DC 20202-2524; (202) 732-1241, 732-1245, 732-1723.

Researches information operations serving the disability field on the national, state, and local levels. Responds to inquiries on a wide range of topics, especially in the areas of Federal funding for programs serving disabled people, Federal legislation affecting the disabled community, and Federal programs benefiting people with disabling conditions. Refers inquirers to appropriate sources of information.

FAMILY INFORMATION Center

National Agricultural Library, Room 304, Department of Agriculture, 10301 Baltimore Boulevard, Beltsville, MD 20705; (301) 344-3719.

Provides information services to professionals concerned with family strengths, well-being, economics, and social environment, and assists them in obtaining current literature regarding the family unit and its individual members. Acquires print and audiovisual resources and develops resource lists and special reference briefs. Document delivery services include lending books and audiovisuals through local or institutional libraries, providing photocopies of journal articles not easily found elsewhere, and helping determine which library owns a particular book, journal, or audiovisual. Open to the public 8:00 a.m. to 4:30 p.m., Monday through Friday.

FOOD AND NUTRITION Information Center (FNIC)

Department of Agriculture, National Agricultural Library, Room 304, 10301 Baltimore Boulevard, Beltsville MD 20705; (301) 344-3719.

Serves the information needs of persons interested in human nutrition, food service management, and food technology. Acquires and lends books and audiovisual materials dealing with these areas of concern. Library open to the public, 8:00 a.m. to 4:30 p.m., Monday through Friday. A 24-hour answering service monitors calls for requests during nonbusiness hours.

National Information Center for Children and Youth with HANDICAPS (NICHCY)

P.O. Box 1492, Washington, DC 20013; (703) 893-6061, (800) 999-5599 (24 hour taped message).

Assists parents, educators, caregivers, advocates, and others working to improve the lives of children and youth with disabilities. Services include personal responses to specific questions, referrals to other organizations/sources of help, and technical assistance to parent and professional groups. Develops and distributes fact sheets on specific disabilities, general information for parents, vocation/transitional issues, special education, and legal rights and advocacy, as well as information on parent support groups and public advocacy.

Office of Disease Prevention and Health Promotion National HEALTH INFORMATION Center (ONHIC)

P.O. Box 1133, Washington, DC 20013-1133; (800) 336-4797, (301) 565-4167.

Helps the public and health professionals locate health information through identification of health information resources, an information and referral system, and publications. Utilizes a database that contains descriptions of health-related organizations to refer inquires to the most appropriate resource. Collection of health reference materials, journals, newsletters, and educational materials is available for use by the public; advance arrangements are recommended. Prepares and distributes publications and directories on health promotion and disease prevention topics.

National HEART, LUNG, AND BLOOD Institute Education Programs Information Center

4733 Bethesda Ave, Suite 530 Bethesda, MD 20814; (301) 951-3260.

Serves as a source of information and materials on cholesterol, smoking, asthma, and high blood pressure – major risk factors for cardiovascular health. Services include dissemination of public education materials, programmatic and scientific information for health professionals, and materials on worksite health, as well as response to information requests. Consumer materials available on asthma, cholesterol, high blood pressure, smoking, chronic cough, heart disease, exercise, stroke, and blood resources. Professional materials available on heart and lung health at the workplace, cholesterol, smoking programs, and blood resources.

National INJURY INFORMATION Clearinghouse

U.S. Consumer Product Safety Commission, 5401 Westbard Avenue, Room 625 Washington, DC 20207; (301) 492-6424.

Collects, investigates, analyzes, and disseminates injury data and information relating to the causes and prevention of death, injury, and illness associated with consumer products. Compiles data obtained from accident investigation reports, consumer complaints/reported incidents, death certificates, news clips, and the CPSC-operated National Electronic Injury Surveillance System (NEISS). Responds to about 6,000 requests for information a year. Publications include statistical analyses of data in the automated files and analyses of hazard and accident patterns.

National KIDNEY AND UROLOGIC Diseases Information Clearinghouse (NKUDIC)

Box NKUDIC 9000 Rockville Pike Bethesda, MD 20892; (301) 468-6345.

Provides education and information on kidney and urologic diseases to patients, professionals, and the public. Makes referrals to other appropriate organizations. Maintains the kidney and urologic diseases subfile of the Combined Health Information Database (CHID). Provides bibliographies on diabetes and kidney disease, audiovisual materials brochures, and fact sheets.

National Institute of MENTAL HEALTH (NIMH)
5600 Fishers Lane, Room 15C-05, Rockville, MD 20857; (301) 443-4513.

Collects scientific, technical, and other information on mental illness and health from the staff and operating components of NIMH and outside sources; classifies, stores, and retrieves information; and answers general inquiries from the public within two weeks. Distributes single copies of NIMH publications at no charge; several consumer publications are in Spanish. Publications list available.

Office of MINORITY HEALTH Resource Center (OMH-RC)
P.O. Box 37337, Washington, DC 20013; (800) 444-6472.

Responds to information requests on minority health, locates sources of technical assistance through the Resource Persons Network, and provides referrals to relevant organizations. Activities concentrate on the minority health priority areas. Bilingual staff members are available to serve Spanish-speaking requesters.

Consumer PRODUCT SAFETY Commission (CPSC)
5401 Westbard Avenue, Room 332, Bethesda, MD 20207; (800) 638-2772 (Consumer Product Safety hotline-national), (800) 638-8270 (hearing impaired-national), (800) 492-8104 (hearing impaired-Maryland).

Maintains the National Injury Information Clearinghouse, conducts investigation into incidents of alleged unsafe/defective products, and establishes product safety standards. Assists consumers in evaluating the comparative safety of products and conducts information and education programs to increase consumer awareness of dangerous products. Operates the National Electronic Injury Surveillance System, which monitors a statistical sample of hospital emergency rooms for injuries associated with consumer products. Maintains free telephone hotline, workdays 8:30 a.m. to 5:00 p.m., to provide information about recalls and about product safety. Hotline operators are on duty to receive reports on product-related accidents, workdays 11:30 a.m. to 4:30 p.m. Publications describe hazards associated with such products as children's toys and electrical products and ways to avoid these hazards.

National REHABILITATION Information Center (NARIC)

8455 Colesville Road, Suite 935, Silver Spring, MD 20910; (301) 588-9284, (800) 34-NARIC.

Supplies publications on disability-related topics, prepares bibliographies tailored to specific requests, and assists in locating answers to questions. Collection includes materials relevant to the rehabilitation of all disability groups, as well as documents relevant to professional and administrative practices and concerns. Collection contains over 300 periodical titles and over 20,000 research reports, books, and audiovisual materials. The public can use the NARIC collection or order materials from the center. Customized literature searches of the NARIC databases are available for nominal fees. Materials available include a periodical holding list and subject catalogue. The center also publishes a directory of rehabilitation librarians and a free quarterly newsletter.

Office on SMOKING AND HEALTH (OSH)

Centers for Disease Control, Department of Health and Human Services, Park Building, Room 1-16, 5600 Fishers Lane, Rockville, MD 20857; (301) 443-1690.

Offers bibliographic and references services to researchers through its Technical Information Center (TIC). Publishes and distributes a number of titles in the field of smoking and health and possesses the computer capability, through its automated search and retrieval system, to generate comprehensive bibliographic printouts on topics of current interest in smoking and health. Epidemiology Branch collects and analyzes numeric data sets that contain significant tobacco use information. Also designs and conducts national surveys on smoking behavior, attitudes, knowledge, and beliefs among adults and teenagers on a periodic basis, and works with other individuals and organizations that are interested in incorporating smoking behavior as part of their survey research activities. Visitors may use the collection, Monday through Friday, 8:30 a.m. to 5:00 p.m. Advance arrangements for visits suggested. Consumer publications on smoking and teenagers, smoking and pregnancy, and smoking cessation are available. Materials for professionals cover cancer, heart diseases, and lung disease associated with smoking.

National Second SURGICAL OPINION Program

Health Care Financing Administration, 200 Independence Avenue SW., Washington, DC 20201; (202) 245-6183 (public information specialist), (800) 638-6833, (800) 492-6603 (Maryland only).

Provides a resource for people faced with the possibility of nonemergency surgery. Sponsors the government's toll-free telephone number to assist callers in locating a surgeon or other specialist. Written requests for information are answered within 14 days. Pamphlet available that poses questions a patient should ask and suggests ways to find a specialist to get a second opinion. Write Surgery, Dept. HHS, Washington, DC 20201.

Toll-Free Numbers for Health Information*

ACQUIRED IMMUNODEFICIENCY SYNDROME (AIDS)

AIDS Clinical Trials Information Service

(800) TRIALS-A. (800)243-7012 TTY/TDD. Provides current information on federally and privately sponsored clinical trials for AIDS patients and others with HIV infection. Sponsored by the Centers for Disease Control, the Food and Drug Administration, the National Institute of Allergy and Infectious Diseases, and the National Library of Medicine. 9 a.m.-7p.m.

National AIDS Information Clearinghouse

(800) 458-5231. Distributes a number of publications on AIDS, including the Surgeon General's report and American Red Cross publications. Refers callers to local information numbers for specific information on AIDS and treatment sources. A service of the U.S. Public Health Service. 9 a.m.-7 p.m.

ALCOHOLISM

Al-Anon Family Group Headquarters

(800) 356-9996. (212) 245-3151 in NY and Canada. Provides printed materials specifically aimed at helping families dealing with the problems of alcoholism. Operates 24 hours.

National Council on Alcoholism

(800) NCA-CALL. Refers to local affiliates and provides written information on alcoholism. Operates 24 hours.

ALZHEIMER'S DISEASE

Alzheimer's Disease and Related Disorders Association

(800) 621-0379. (800) 572-6037 in IL. Refers to local chapters and support groups. Offers information on publications available from the association. 9 a.m.-5 p.m. (central time)

* Reprinted by permission. National Health Information Center.

Brookdale Center on Aging - Alzheimer's Respite Line

(800) 648-COPE for placing orders. Provides information packets to assist health professionals and family caregivers in setting up community respite centers for patients and their families. A service of the Brookdale Foundation and Hunter College. Orders may be placed 24 hours.

ARTHRITIS

Arthritis Foundation Information Line

(800) 283-7800. Provides publications and information about arthritis and referrals to local organizations. 9 a.m.-7 p.m.

CANCER

Cancer Information Service (CIS)

(800) 4-CANCER. (800) 524-1234 in Oahu, HI (neighbor islands call collect). (800) 638-6070 in AK. Answers cancer-related questions from the public, cancer patients and families, and health professionals. Spanish-speaking staff members are available to callers from the following areas: CA, FL, GA, IL, northern NJ, New York City, and TX. A service of the National Cancer Institute. 9 a.m.-10 p.m.; 10 a.m.-6 p.m. Saturday.

Cancer Response Line

(800) ACS-2345. Provides publications and information about cancer and coping with cancer. Refers callers to local chapters of the American Cancer Society for support services. A service of the American Cancer Society. 8:30 a.m.-4:30 p.m.

Y-Me Breast Cancer Support Program

(800) 221-2141. (312) 799-8228 in IL. Provides breast cancer patients with presurgery counseling, treatment information, peer support, self-help counseling, and patient literature; also makes referrals according to guidelines from its medical advisory board. 9 a.m.-5 p.m. (central time); local number operates 24 hours.

CYSTIC FIBROSIS

Cystic Fibrosis Foundation
(800) 344-4823. (301) 951-4422 in MD. Responds to patient and family questions and offers literature. Provides referrals to local clinics. 8:30 a.m.-5:30 p.m.

DIABETES

American Diabetes Association
(800) ADA-DISC. (703) 549-1500 in VA and DC metro area. Provides free literature, a newsletter, information on health education, and refers to local affiliates for support group assistance. 8:30 a.m.-5 p.m.

DOWN'S SYNDROME

National Down's Syndrome Congress
(800) 232-6372. (312) 823-7550 in IL. Answers questions from parents about health concerns. Refers to local organizations. 9 a.m.-5 p.m. (central time).

National Down's Syndrome Society Hotline
(800) 221-4602. (212) 460-9330 in NY. Offers information on Down's syndrome and gives referrals to local programs for the newborn. Provides free information packet upon request. 9 a.m-5 p.m.

DRUG ABUSE

National Cocaine Hotline
(800) COC-AINE. Answers questions on the health risks of cocaine to cocaine users, their friends and families. Provides referrals to drug rehabilitation centers. A service of the Psychiatric Institute of America. Operates 24 hours.

EATING DISORDERS

Bulimia Anorexia Self-Help
(800) 227-4785. Provides information on bulimia, anorexia, depression, anxiety, and phobias. 8:30 a.m.-5 p.m. (central

time). For 24-hour crisis intervention and information use the Bulimia Anorexia Self-Help Crisis Line: (800) 762-3334.

FITNESS

Aerobics and Fitness Foundation
(800) BE FIT 86. Answers questions from the public regarding safe and effective exercise programs and practices. 10 a.m.-5 p.m. (Pacific time).

FOOD SAFETY

Meat and Poultry Hotline
(800) 535-4555. Provides safety hints on proper handling preparation, storage, and cooking of meat, poultry, and eggs. Sponsored by the U.S. Department of Agriculture. 10 a.m.-4 p.m.

GENERAL HEALTH

ODPHP National Health Information Center
(800) 336-4797. (301) 565-4167 in DC metro area. Provides a central source of information and referral for health questions from health educators, health professionals, and the general public. Spanish-speaking staff available. A service of the Office of Disease Prevention and Health Promotion, U.S. Department of Health and Human Services. 9 a.m-5 p.m.

GLAUCOMA

Foundation for Glaucoma Research
(800) 245-3005. (415) 986-3162. Provides consumer information and funds biomedical research. 8:30 a.m.-6 p.m.

HANDICAPPING CONDITIONS
see also HEARING AND SPEECH

The Epilepsy Foundation of America
(800) EFA-1000. (301) 459-3700 in MD. (800) 492-2523 Baltimore. Provides information on epilepsy and makes referrals to local chapters. 9 a.m.-5 p.m.

HEALTH Resource Center

(800) 544-3284. (202) 939-9320 in DC. Provides information on postsecondary education for the handicapped and on learning disabilities. 9 a.m-5 p.m.

IBM National Support Center for Persons with Disabilities

(800) IBM-2133 Voice/TDD. Responds to requests for information on how computers can help people with vision and hearing problems, speech impairments, learning disabilities, mental retardation, and mobility problems. It is a clearinghouse for information on all types of available equipment and staff will assess an individual's needs and make appropriate referrals. 8:30 a.m.-5 p.m.

Library of Congress National Library Services for the Blind and Physically Handicapped

(800) 424-8567. (202) 707-5100 in DC. Provides both audio and Braille formats for the blind and physically handicapped, or anyone who is unable to read print for any reason, through a network of state libraries. 8 a.m.-4:30 p.m.

National Information System for Health Related Services (NIS)

(800) 922-9234. (800) 922-1107 in SC. Makes referrals to support groups and sources of financial, medical and legal assistance for developmentally disabled and chronically ill children up to age 21. 8:30 a.m.-5 p.m.

National Rehabilitation Information Center

(800) 34-NARIC. (301) 588-9284 in MD. Provides rehabilitation information on assistive devices and disseminates other rehabilitation-related information. 8 a.m.-8 p.m.

HEADACHE

National Headache Foundation

(800) 843-2256. (800) 523-8858 in IL. Offers membership information and sends literature on headaches and treatment. 9 a.m.-5 p.m. (central time)

HEARING AND SPEECH

Dial A Hearing Test

(800) 222-EARS. (800) 345-EARS in PA. Answers questions on hearing problems and makes referrals to local numbers for a two-minutes hearing test, as well as ear, nose, and throat specialists. Also makes referrals to organizations that have information on ear-related problems, including questions on broken hearing aids. 9 a.m.-6 p.m.

Hearing Helpline

(800) 424-8576. (800) EAR-WELL. (703) 642-0580 in VA. Provides information on better hearing and preventing deafness. Materials are mailed on request. A service of the Better Hearing Institute. 9 a.m.-5 p.m.

National Association for Hearing and Speech Action Line

(800) 638-8255. (301) 897-0039 in HI, AK, and MD (call collect). Offers information and distributes materials on hearing aids and pathologists and audiologists certified by the American Speech-Language-Hearing Association. 8:30 a.m.-4:30 p.m.

National Hearing Aid Helpline

(800) 521-5247. (313) 478-2610 in MI. Provides information and distributes a directory of hearing aid specialists certified by the National Hearing Aid Society. 9 a.m.-5 p.m.

Tele-Consumer Hotline

(800) 332-1124 Voice/TDD. (202) 223-4371 in DC. Provides information about relay services between people with hearing or speech impairments and people without communication impairment; also helps all disabled individuals locate communication equipment. Spanish language assistance available. 9 a.m.-5 p.m.

HOSPICE CARE

Hospice Education Institute Hospicelink

(800) 331-1620. (203) 767-1620 in CT. Offers general information about hospice care and makes referrals to local

programs. Does not offer medical advice or personal counseling. 9 a.m.-5 p.m.

HOSPITAL CARE

Hill-Burton Hospital Free Care

(800) 638-0742. (800) 492-0359 in MD. Provides information on hospitals and other health facilities participating in the Hill-Burton Hospital Free Care Program. A service of the Bureau of Resources Development, U.S. Department of Health and Human Services. 9:30 a.m.-5:30 p.m. or leave recorded message 24 hours.

IMPOTENCE

Recovery of Male Potency

(800) 835-7667. (313) 357-1216 in MI. Provides referrals to self-help support groups associated with ROMP and other agencies. Distributes information packet. A service of Grace Hospital, Detroit, MI, and affiliated with 23 hospitals nationwide. 8 a.m.-4:30 p.m.

INCOME TAX

Federal Internal Revenue Service for TDD Users

(800) 428-4732 TDD. (800) 382-4059 TDD in IN. (800) 424-1040 Voice. Answers questions on Federal income tax, including medical deductions for the cost of tele-communications devices for the deaf (TDDs), hearing aids, trained hearing-ear dogs, and sending deaf children to special schools. Accepts orders for publications on tax information for handicapped and disabled individuals, and other free IRS publications. 8:30 a.m.-4:30 p.m.

LIVER DISEASES

American Liver Foundation

(800) 232-0179. (201) 256-2550 in NJ. Provides information including fact sheets, and making physician and support group referrals. 8:30 a.m.-4:30 p.m.

LUNG DISEASES

Asthma Information Line

(800) 822-ASMA. Provides written materials on asthma and allergies. A service of the American Academy of Allergy and Immunology. Operates 24 hours.

Lung Line National Asthma Center

(800) 222-5864. (303) 355-LUNG in Denver. Answers questions about asthma, emphysema, chronic bronchitis, allergies, juvenile rheumatoid arthritis, smoking, and other respiratory and immune system disorders. Questions answered by registered nurses. A service of the National Jewish Center for Immunology and Respiratory Medicine. 8 a.m.-5 p.m. (mountain time).

LUPUS

Lupus Foundation of America

(800) 558-0121. (202) 328-4550 in DC. Answers basic questions about the disease and provides health professionals and patients and their families with information and literature. Refers to local affiliates. 9 a.m.-5 p.m.

Terri Gotthelf Lupus Research Institute

(800) 82-LUPUS. (203) 852-0120 in CT. Offers information and distributes materials on lupus, including a list of centers that conduct research and provide health services to lupus patients. 9 a.m.-7 p.m.

MEDICARE/MEDICAID

DHHS Inspector General's Hotline

(800) 368-5779. (301) 965-5953 in MD. Handles complaints regarding fraud, waste, and abuse of government funds, including Medicare, Medicaid, and Social Security. Assists people who have been overbilled or billed for services not rendered. 10 a.m.-4 p.m. or leave recorded message 24 hours.

MENTAL HEALTH

American Mental Health Fund

(800) 433-5959. (800) 826-2336 in IL. Provides a 24-hour recorded message for callers to request the AMHF pamphlet that includes general information about the organization and mental health and warning signs of mental illness.

National Foundation for Depressive Illness

(800) 248-4344. A 24-hour recorded message describes symptoms of depression and gives an address for more information and physician referral.

MINORITY HEALTH

Office of Minority Health Resource Center

(800) 444-6472. Responds to consumer and professional inquiries on minority health related topics by distributing materials, providing referrals to appropriate sources, and identifying sources of technical assistance. Spanish-speaking staff available. 9 a.m.-5 p.m.

MULTIPLE SCLEROSIS

National Multiple Sclerosis Society

(800) 624-8236. Provides a 24-hour recording for callers to request information and leave name and address. To speak to a staff member, call (800) 227-3166. 11 a.m.-6 p.m.

ORGAN DONATION
see also RETINITIS PIGMENTOSA and UROLOGICAL DISORDERS

The Living Bank

(800) 528-2971. (713) 528-2971 in TX. Operates a registry and referral service for people wanting to commit their tissues, bones, or vital organs to transplantation or research. Informs the public about organ donation and transplantation. Operates 24 hours.

PARALYSIS AND SPINAL CORD INJURY
see also HANDICAPPING CONDITIONS

American Paralysis Association
(800) 225-0292. (201) 379-2690 in NJ. Answers questions about research on head and spinal injuries. Raises money to fund research to find a cure for paralysis caused by spinal and head injuries or stroke. 9 a.m.-5 p.m.

APA Spinal Cord Injury Hotline
(800) 526-3456. Offers literature on spinal cord injuries and makes referrals to organizations and support groups. Sponsored by the American Paralysis Association. 9 a.m.-4:30 p.m.

National Spinal Cord Injury Association
(800) 962-9629. (617) 935-2722 in MA. Provides peer counseling to those suffering from spinal cord injuries and makes referrals to local chapters and other organizations. Produces the National Resource Directory that deals with topics helpful to handicapped individuals. 9 a.m.-5 p.m.

PARKINSON'S DISEASE

National Parkinson Foundation
(800) 327-4545. (800) 433-7022 in FL. (305) 547-6666 in Miami. Answers questions about the disease: staffed by nurses. Also makes physician referrals and provides written materials. 8 a.m.-5 p.m.

Parkinson's Education Program
(800) 344-7872. (714) 640-0218 in CA. Provides materials such as newsletters, a glossary of definitions, a videotape, and publications catalogues. Offers patient-support group information and physician referrals. Operates 24 hours.

RARE DISORDERS

American Leprosy Missions (Hansen's Disease)
(800) 543-3131. (201) 794-8650 in NJ. Answers questions and distributes materials on the disease. 8:30 a.m.-5 p.m.

Cooley's Anemia Foundation

(800) 221-3571. (212) 598-0911 in NY. Provides information on patient care, research, fundraising, patient-support groups, and research grants. Makes referrals to local chapters. 9 a.m.-5 p.m.

Cornelia De Lange Syndrome Foundation

(800) 223-8355. (203) 693-0159 in CT. Provides a variety of materials for families, friends, and professionals about this syndrome. 9 a.m.-5 p.m. or leave recorded message 24 hours.

Histiocytosis Association of America

(800) 548-2758. (609) 881-4911 in NJ. Offers printed material and emotional support for persons with histiocytosis. 9 a.m.-5 p.m.

National Lymphedema Network

(800) 541-3259. Provides information on lymphedema and other venous disorders. Gives referrals to treatment centers. 8 a.m.-6 p.m. (Pacific time).

National Neurofibromatosis Foundation

(800) 323-7938. (212) 460-8980 in NY. Responds to inquiries from health professionals and patients and families. Makes referrals to physicians on clinical advisory board. 9 a.m.-5 p.m.

Tourette's Syndrome Association

(800) 237-0717. (718) 224-2999 in NY. Provides a 24-hour recording for callers to request information and leave name and address. To speak with a staff member, call the local number between 9 a.m.-5 p.m.

United Scleroderma Foundation

(800) 722-HOPE. (408) 728-2202 in CA. Provides lists of publications, chapters throughout the United States, and general information. 8 a.m.-5 p.m. (Pacific time).

RETINITIS PIGMENTOSA

National Retinitis Pigmentosa Foundation
(800) 638-2300. (301) 225-9400 in MD. Responds to questions and makes available an information packet on the disease. Covers genetics, current research, and retina donor programs. 8:30 a.m.-5 p.m.

REYE'S SYNDROME

National Reye's Syndrome Foundation
(800) 233-7393. (800) 231-7393 in OH. Provides general information and referrals to families for peer counseling. 8:30 a.m.-5 p.m. (central time).

SAFETY
see also CHEMICAL PRODUCTS

Consumer Product Safety Commission
(800) 638-CPSC. (800) 638-8270 TDD. (800) 492-8104 TDD in MD. Provides 24-hour recording on consumer product safety, including product hazards and product defects and injuries sustained in using products. Covers only products used in and around the home, excluding automobiles, foods, drugs, cosmetics, boats, and firearms.

SICKLE CELL DISEASE

National Association for Sickle Cell Disease
(800) 421-8453. (213) 936-7205 in CA. Offers genetic counseling and an information packet. 8:30 a.m.-5:30 p.m. (Pacific time).

SPINA BIFIDA

Spina Bifida Information and Referral
(800) 621-3141. (301) 770-7222 in MD. Provides information to consumers and health professionals and referrals to local chapters. A service of the Spina Bifida Association of America. 9 a.m.-5 p.m.

UROLOGICAL DISORDERS

American Kidney Fund

(800) 638-8299. (800) 492-8361 in MD. Grants financial assistance to kidney patients who are unable to pay treatment-related costs. Also provides information on organ donations and kidney-related diseases. 8 a.m.-5 p.m.

VISION

American Council of the Blind

(800) 424-8666. (202) 393-3666 in DC. Offers information on blindness. Provides referrals to clinics, rehabilitation organizations, research centers, and local chapters. Also published resource lists. 9 a.m.-5:30 p.m.

American Foundation for the Blind (AFB)

(800) 232-5463. (212) 620-2147 in NY. Gives information on visual impairments and blindness and on AFB services, products, and publications. 8:30 a.m.-4:30 p.m.

National Center for Sight

(800) 221-3004. Provides information on a broad range of eye health and safety topics. Sponsored by the National Society to Prevent Blindness. 9 a.m.-4 p.m. (central time).

National Eye Care Project Helpline

(800) 222-EYES. Offers information on free eye examination for the financially disadvantaged who are at least 65 years old, American citizens, and who have not seen an ophthalmologist in three years. 8 a.m.-5 p.m. (Pacific time).

WOMEN

Endometriosis Association

(800) 992-ENDO. (414) 962-8972 in WI. Provides a 24-hour recording for callers to request information and leave name and address.

Additional Association Services

The Visiting Nurses Association of America
3801 East Florida Avenue, Suite 806, Denver, Colorado, 80210, (800) 426-2547.

National Stroke Association
1420 Ogden Street, Denver, Colorado, 80218. (303) 839-1992.

American Association of Retired Persons
601 E Street, NE, Washington, D.C., 20049

American Health Care Association
5615 West Cermak Road, Cicero, Illinois, 60650 or 1201 L Street, NW, Washington DC. 20005-4014.

National Association of Home Care
519 C Street NE, Washington, D.C., 20002-5809

American Heart Association National Center
7320 Greenville Avenue, Dallas, Texas. 75231

American Diabetes Association
(Diabetes Information Service Center) 1660 Duke Street. Alexandia, Virginia 22314. (800) ADA-DISC.

National Multiple Sclerosis Society
205 East 42 Street. New York, NY 10017-5706 (800) 624-8236.

SERVICES FOR THE DEAF

National Center for Law and the Deaf
800 Florida Avenue, Washington, DC, 20002.

Registry of Interpreters for the Deaf
51 Monroe Street, Rockville, NY, 20950

Captioning for the Deaf
500 Park Street North, St. Petersburg, Florida 33709

Telecommunications for the Deaf, Inc.
814 Thayer Avenue, Silver Springs, Maryland, 20910.

National Hearing Aid Society
24261 Grand River, Detroit, Michigan, 48219.

Dogs of the Deaf
10175 Wheeler Road, Central Point, Oregon 97502

Magazines, Publications, Catalogues

Independent Living
Equal Opportunity Publications. 44 Broadway, Greenlawn, NY 11740-1316. (516) 261-9086. A magazine with articles about issues and problems concerning people with disabilities. Includes equipment, supplies, services for disabled people.

Continuing Care
Stevens Publishing Company. 225 North New Road, Waco, Texas 76710. Catalogue of home care products for people with disabilities.

Northcoast Medical, Inc.
187 Stauffen Blvd., San Jose, California, 95125-1042. A catalogue of adaptive equipment for people with physical disabilities.

Adaptability
P.O. Box 515. Colchester, Connecticut, 06415-0515. (800) 243-9232. A catalogue of assistive devices and equipment to improve independent living.

Fashion Able for Better Living
5 Crescent Avenue, Box S Rocky Hill, New Jersey 08553. (609) 921-2563. A catalogue containing reading, writing , and phone aids; footcare supplies; daily living and comfort aids, and beauty and health supplies.

Comfortably Yours
61 West Hunter Avenue, Maywood, New Jersey, 07607 (201) 368-0400. A wide range of clothing and undergarments, support garments, shoes, health & exercise and houseware supplies for people with reduced or limited physical capacity.

J.C. Penny's Mail Order Catalogue of Adaptive Clothing
Available from your local J.C. Penny's store. For women only.

Enrichment for Better Living
145 Tower Drive, P.O. Box 579 Hinsdale, Illinois 60521 (800) 323-5547. A catalogue featuring a wide range of supplies and equipment for meal preparation, eating, dressing, bathing, and leisure activities.

LS and S Group. Inc.
P.O. Box 673, Northbrook, Illinois 60065. (800) 468-4789. Specializing in products for the visually impaired.

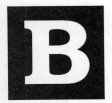

Medicare
and Medicaid

As you attempt to find more information about financing for health care, you may find that this is quite a confusing process. This is a time full of stress and pressures in which you are learning new things; the burden of large medical bills and coordinating payments certainly does not ease your burden. Below are descriptions of medicare and medicaid programs, what they cover, who is eligible, and how you can get more specific information and help.

Medicare

Medicare is a medical insurance program, and is the largest national health care expenditure. Medicare was enacted on July 30, 1965 as Title XVIII of the Social Security Act and expanded by the 1972 Amendments to the Social Security Act. There have been numerous other changes in medicare law during the 1980s through the Omnibus Budget Reconciliation Act and deficit reduction legislation.

The medicare program consists of two parts. Part A, the Hospital Insurance Program, covers hospital inpatient, skilled nursing facility, and hospice care. Part A is provided automatically for those who are eligible and pays for all covered services.

Part B, the Supplemental Medical Insurance Program, covers hospital outpatient, physicians, home health, comprehensive outpatient rehabilitation facilities, and other professional services. Part B may be purchased for a monthly premium by those who are already eligible for Part A. After a beneficiary meets an annual deductible, Part B covers 80% of costs for approved services.

Eligibility for medicare begins when a person turns 65 years old. People who are eligible must also be eligible for monthly Social Security retirement or survivor benefits, or be Railroad Retirement beneficiaries, or merchant seamen. People who are over 65 years old but who do not fit into this profile have the option to purchase Part A and B coverage. People under 65 may also be eligible if they have been entitled to Social Security or Railroad Retirement benefits because of a disability for 24 consecutive months. Also people with end stage renal disease are eligible for medicare if they are entitled to other Social Security benefits or if they are spouses or dependents of insured people.

To find more information about the medicare program, go to your nearest Social Security office or call the Health Care Financing Administration, which is a division of the Department of Health and Human Services, and which will be listed in your phone book.

Medicaid

Medicaid is an assistance program, and is the second largest national health care expenditure. This is a joint federal and state program which was enacted in 1966 as Title XIX of the Social Security Act. The medicaid program varies slightly from state to state, but basically its purpose is to provide health care assistance to the poor and the medically indigent.

Medicaid coverage will vary from state to state, but in all states the following services are covered: inpatient hospital care, outpatient hospital services, other laboratory procedures, skilled nursing facilities services, physician services, screening and treatment for young children, home health care services, family planning services, and rural health care clinic services.

Medicaid eligibility will vary from state to state, but beneficiaries generally include some people who are 65 or older, people who are blind or have some other disability, members of poor families with dependent children, and certain pregnant women.

As medicaid programs can be so variable, it is best to contact your state or local welfare office, or the Health Care Financing Administration. Both of these agencies will be listed in your phone book.

Be prepared with financial information, social security number, and medical condition and needs of the potential beneficiary when you call these offices for information on either program. Having specific questions in mind will also be beneficial if you are making phone contact only. If you are in need of more specific information, you may have to visit the local offices, and in that case, again be prepared with the necessary information.

Managing the medical bills associated with lengthy illnesses and home care will never be easy, but with a little information, patience, and perseverance you will be able to do quite well. Remember to contact the social worker at the hospital or home health care agency for extra assistance; these people are very adept at managing these systems and helping with the appropriate paperwork.

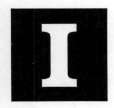

Index

Page numbers listed in **boldface** refer to pages with illustrations.